Y0-BSZL-922

The Clinical Management
of Anxiety Disorders

The Clinical Management
of Anxiety Disorders

EDITED BY

William Coryell, M.D.

George Winokur, M.D.

Department of Psychiatry
University of Iowa
College of Medicine

New York   Oxford
OXFORD UNIVERSITY PRESS
1991

Oxford University Press

Oxford New York Toronto
Delhi Bombay Calcutta Madras Karachi
Petaling Jaya Singapore Hong Kong Tokyo
Nairobi Dar es Salaam Cape Town
Melbourne Auckland

and associated companies in
Berlin Ibadan

Copyright © 1991 by Oxford University Press, Inc.

Published by Oxford University Press, Inc.,
200 Madison Avenue, New York, New York 10016

Oxford is a registered trademark of Oxford University Press

All rights reserved. No part of this publication may be reproduced,
stored in a retrieval system, or transmitted, in any form or by any means,
electronic, mechanical, photocopying, recording, or otherwise,
without the prior permission of Oxford University Press.

Library of Congress Cataloging-in-Publication Data
The clinical management of anxiety disorders / edited by
William Coryell, George Winokur.
p. cm.
Includes bibliographical references.
Includes index.
ISBN 0-19-505953-0
1. Anxiety—Treatment. I. Coryell, William
II. Winokur, George.
[DNLM: 1. Anxiety Disorders—therapy. WM 172 C6418]
RC531.C58 1991
616.85′223—dc20
DNLM/DLC   90-7261 CIP

For information about our audio products, write us at:
Newbridge Book Clubs, 3000 Cindel Drive, Delran, NJ 08370

9 8 7 6 5 4 3 2 1

Printed in the United States of America
on acid-free paper

Preface

The anxiety disorders are both disabling and prevalent. Research into treatment has been correspondingly vigorous, especially in the past decade. The researchers, however, have been a varied group. Behaviorists, psychopharmacologists, and cognitive therapists have approached treatment issues with individual orientations, interests, and preconceptions. The resulting literature, vital to the informed clinician, is scattered and unwieldy.

Of course, texts are available to distill certain broad areas. Generally, these cover one type of therapy in depth or they superficially cover many therapies in many disorders. There seems to be a clear place for a text that describes all empirically founded treatment with a focus on the anxiety disorders.

In response, we have targeted a book for clinicians who need both an overview and a thorough bibliography. Sections are organized by diagnosis and, within diagnoses, by treatment. The authors have heavily referenced their text throughout to assist readers who require more depth. Cognitive and behavioral strategies are given special attention—they have their own chapters subdivided by diagnoses. At the risk of some redundancy, the subsequent chapters also describe psychotherapeutic approaches and then compare and integrate these with psychopharmacotherapies. The book concludes with a condensation and synthesis of all therapies across all anxiety disorders. We have attempted to end up with a book that will be useful as a manual of the anxiety disorders and an asset to the clinician who is managing patients with these problems.

Contents

Contributors

James C. Ballenger, M.D., Ph.D.
Department of Psychiatry and
  Behavioral Sciences
Medical University of
  South Carolina
College of Medicine
Charleston, South Carolina 29425

Wayne A. Bowers, Ph.D.
Department of Medicine
University of Iowa
College of Medicine
Iowa City, Iowa 52242

William Coryell, M.D.
Department of Psychiatry
University of Iowa
College of Medicine
Iowa City, Iowa 52242

Jonathan Davidson, M.D.
Duke University Medical Center
John Umstead Hospital
Butner, North Carolina 27509

Michael Gelder, Professor
Department of Psychiatry
University of Oxford
The Warneford Hospital
Oxford, England OX3 7JX

Rudolf Hoehn-Saric, M.D.
Department of Psychiatry
The Johns Hopkins University
School of Medicine
Baltimore, Maryland 21205

Michael A. Jenike, M.D.
Department of Psychiatry
Harvard Medical School
Boston, Massachusetts 02115

Michael R. Liebowitz, M.D.
Department of Psychiatry
Columbia University
College of Physicians
  and Surgeons
New York, New York 10032

Daniel R. McLeod, Ph.D.
Department of Psychiatry
The Johns Hopkins University
School of Medicine
Baltimore, Maryland 21205

Russell Noyes, Jr., M.D.
Department of Psychiatry
University of Iowa
College of Medicine
Iowa City, Iowa 52242

George Winokur, M.D.
Department of Psychiatry
University of Iowa
College of Medicine
Iowa City, Iowa 52242

The Clinical Management
of Anxiety Disorders

1

Anxiety Disorders: The Magnitude of the Problem

GEORGE WINOKUR AND WILLIAM CORYELL

Like other terms in clinical psychiatry, such as "depression," "hysteria," and "borderline," "anxiety" suffers from multiple meanings. To the dynamic psychologist, anxiety is a drive state occurring as a result of intrapsychic conflict, the relief of which is highly to be desired by the person. To the dictionary buff, it is a state of uneasiness much akin to fear and apprehension. To the clinician, however, anxiety connotes a disorder or illness or, at the very least, a syndrome that has certain symptoms. It is the definition of anxiety as a disorder that concerns us in this book. Patients with such disorders appear in the offices of clinicians and demand to be treated for them. Major questions are how many anxiety disorders can be diagnosed and how frequently they are seen in various kinds of settings.

Commonly used diagnostic criteria (DSM III-R, 1987) define seven different types of anxiety disorders. The thread that connects them is the presence of anxiety and avoidance behaviors as predominant features. Table 1–1 presents features that are seen in the various types of anxiety disorders.

How many of these syndromes deserve to be considered separate illnesses is open to question. Considerable clinical, follow-up, and family data support the categories of panic disorder with or without agoraphobia, obsessional disorders, and simple phobias. The most distinct group is post-traumatic stress disorder, which is different from the others because its definition encompasses a special experiential factor. Agoraphobia by itself, social phobia, and generalized anxiety disorder are probably best left for more research in order to achieve better understanding of their place or even possibly their existence.

That these diagnoses may not always be valid is documented by a number of studies. Tyrer and his colleagues (1987) evaluated the symptoms of anxiety, panic, depression, hypochondriasis, and phobias over a two-year period and found considerable temporal variability of anxiety and depressive symptoms that were poorly related to the diagnosis. Pho-

Table 1–1 Common Features in the Anxiety Disorders

	Panic Disorder	Agoraphobia	Social Phobia	Simple Phobia	OBS Comp	PTSD	GAD
Panic attacks	+*	–	±	±			±
Agoraphobia	*	+*		±			–
Fear of embarrassment in social situations	–	+*	+*	+			–
Avoidance of situations	±	+	+	+	±	+	–
Recognizes illness is unreasonable		–	+	+	+		–
Recurrent and persistent ideas	–	–	–	–	+*		–
Repetitive behaviors	–	–	–	–	+*		–
Motor, tension, autonomic hyperactivity, vigilance	+	+	+	+		+	+*
Generalized nervousness	+				+	+	+*
Secondary depression	+				+	+	+
Fear of circumscribed situations				+*			
Intense fear, secondary to distressing event						+*	
Re-experiencing the event						+*	
Impulsive behavior, anger attacks						+	

*Criteria symptoms; PTSD = Post-traumatic stress disorder; obs-comp = Obsessive-compulsive disorder; GAD = generalized anxiety disorder bic symptoms, on the other hand, remained relatively consistent over time. The authors suggested that classification of neurotic disorders based on presenting anxiety and depressive symptoms was unsatisfactory; many patients could be classified as having a single mixed disorder. This comment does not take into account the possible usefulness of the primary-secondary distinction, except to cite Woodruff et al. (1967), who gave a definition of secondary depression.

In any event, the temporal instability of the symptoms, and the question of what came first and what transpired afterward, create a classification problem. Tyrer (1986) also suggests that whatever classification is ultimately adopted, panic disorder probably will not persist as a separate entity, and the best possible solution would be to combine the so-called anxiety disorders under the rubric of "genetic neurotic syndrome." This would encompass conditions that have important genetic components, show priority of different symptoms at different times, and are associated with personality traits of dependency.

Noyes et al. (1987) published data from a family study of generalized anxiety disorder that compound the problem of diagnosis. They found that the frequency of generalized anxiety disorder was higher among first-degree relatives of probands with generalized anxiety than among relatives of control subjects, but was not higher than in relatives with panic disorder or agoraphobia. Alternatively, panic disorder was higher in relatives of probands with panic disorder than among control relatives, but was not higher among relatives of generalized anxiety probands compared to control relatives. Relatives of probands with generalized anxiety who had the same disorder had a mild stress-related illness. The authors concluded that the separation of generalized anxiety disorder and panic disorder was confirmed, but that a separation between generalized anxiety and adjustment disorders was not supported by the data.

Though there is marked uncertainty about the specificity of diagnosis and the existence of distinct anxiety disorders, the frequency with which these disorders is encountered is clear.

Early estimates of the prevalence of anxiety disorders were made in clinical settings (Wheeler et al., 1950). Thus, anxiety states, which were then called "neurocirculatory asthenias" or "anxiety neuroses," were often seen in a cardiologist's office, mainly because the patient's complaints were those of "functional" heart symptoms. Likewise, the psychological aspects of the anxiety disorders, such as intense apprehension and the fear of dying, sometimes brought patients to psychiatric clinics. Among the interesting observations of that period was the finding that anxiety disorders were uncommon among longshoremen and more common among people with white-collar jobs. Longshoremen do heavy work on the docks that would not be appealing to anxiety-disordered patients or to people with fatigue and a feeling that they might have heart problems. However, evaluations of the epidemiology of the anxiety disorders were incomplete until the advent of population studies in psychiatry.

Table 1–2   Lifetime Prevalence Rates in ECA Study

	Both Sexes	*Males*	*Females*
Phobia	7.8(0.4)–23.3(0.8)		
Panic	1.4(0.2)–1.5(0.3)	0.6(0.2)–1.2(0.3)	1.6(0.3)–2.1(0.4)
Obsessive-compulsive	1.9(0.3)–3.0(0.3)	1.1(0.3)–2.6(0.6)	2.6(0.5)–3.3(0.5)
Agoraphobia		1.5(0.3)–5.2(0.6)	5.3(0.5)–12.5(1.0)
Simple phobia		3.8(0.5)–14.5(1.1)	8.5(0.7)–25.9(1.2)

The most recent and thorough study of anxiety disorders in the general population was part of the Epidemiologic Catchment Area study (ECA). Table 1–2 presents the results of this study, summarizing the lifetime prevalence of specific anxiety disorders in three sites (St. Louis, New Haven, and Baltimore). The lifetime prevalence figures are calculated as the proportion of persons in a representative sample of the population who have ever experienced that disorder up to the date of assessment (Robins et al., 1984). Phobias are obviously seen in a large proportion of the population; in one center, they were found in almost one-quarter of the subjects. Summing the rates of phobia, panic disorder, and obsessive-compulsive disorder in both sexes, it can be concluded that 11.1 to 27.8 percent of the population will have at least one of these conditions. In the ECA study, the other conditions that were seen most commonly were substance abuse and the affective disorders.

From the individual diagnoses, it is clear that panic disorder, obsessive-compulsive disorder, agoraphobia, and social phobia are all more common in women than in men.

There were marked intersite differences among the collaborating centers. Baltimore showed a high lifetime prevalence of agoraphobia and simple phobia, and was significantly higher for obsessive-compulsive disorder than St. Louis.

By and large, race made little difference, though there were significantly higher rates for simple phobias among blacks in Baltimore and St. Louis (but not in New Haven). Education was inversely related to the rates of simple phobias and agoraphobia in the study. College graduates showed significantly lower rates of agoraphobia and simple phobia than noncollege graduates. These differences in education were not found in obsessive-compulsive disorder.

Though variations were associated with certain demographic factors (e.g., location, sex), the striking finding was the high frequency of anxiety disorders in the general population. The study also yielded data on six-month prevalence rates in the same three communities (Meyers et al., 1984). For the six-month period immediately preceding the interview, the prevalence rates for panic disorder in men were 0.3 to 0.8 percent, and in women they were 0.9 to 1.2 percent. For obsessive-compulsive disorder, the six-month prevalence rates were 0.9 to 1.9 percent in men and 1.7 to 2.2 percent in women.

Table 1–3 Post-Traumatic Stress Disorder in the General Population

	Men	Women
Number of people interviewed	965	1,528
Cases/1000 due to any trauma	5.0	13.0
Cases/1000 due to combat	3.3	0.0
Cases/1000 due to physical attack	0.0	4.6
Cases/1000 due to seeing someone hurt or die	1.7	1.4

Post-traumatic stress disorder was also studied in one of the ECA sites, namely, St. Louis (Helzer et al., 1987). The rates found in this study are presented in Table 1–3. Although meeting the full diagnostic criteria for the disorder was unusual, experiencing some symptoms of post-traumatic stress disorder after trauma was not uncommon. This was true of both men (15 percent) and women (16 percent). For men, combat was the most likely cause of symptoms; for women, the common causes were physical attack, seeing somebody hurt or die, physical threat, or a close call. The duration varied. Combat symptoms were particularly long-lived; one-half of the men had had them for more than three years. For the women, physical attack was associated with long-lasting symptoms.

It might be concluded that post-traumatic stress disorder is not seen in the population at very high frequencies. The prevalence of a history of post-traumatic stress disorder was 1 percent in the total population, about 3.5 percent in civilians exposed to physical attack, and 3.5 percent in Vietnam veterans who were not wounded and 20 percent in veterans who were wounded. These epidemiological findings go a long way to suggest certain populations that are at special risk and could be identified for treatment. The condition is often associated with behavioral problems in childhood.

Many studies suggest that anxiety disorders run in families. Table 1–4 presents the results of one family study (Noyes et al., 1987). The findings suggest a genetic factor in the etiology of the anxiety disorders. In regard to practice and treatment, the data suggest that by taking a family history, the clinician may uncover many individuals who could benefit from treatment.

Not always do these syndromes or disorders necessitate treatment, and not always do people seek help for them. In a twenty-year follow-up study of patients with anxiety neuroses (neurocirculatory asthenia) who were diagnosed in a cardiologist's office before 1928, 12 percent were well and 35 percent were much improved at the time of follow-up (Wheeler et al., 1950). However, 53 percent were unimproved or disabled. Treatment for these patients in the 1920s was rudimentary. These data are important because they are indicative of the natural history of the disease before the modern era of treatment. In a more recent study, 24–31 percent of persons diagnosed as having anxiety disorders in the general population in the

Table 1–4 Anxiety Disorders in Primary Relatives of Controls and Anxiety Disorder Patients

	Controls	Generalized (N=20)	Panic (N=20)	Agoraphobia (N=40)	P (N=40)
Number of relatives	113	123	241	256	
Proportion of relatives ill with:					
All anxiety disorders	13.3%	30.1%	25.7%	27.7%	.05
Panic disorder	3.5%	4.1%	14.9%	7.0%	.001
Agoraphobia	3.5%	3.3%	1.7%	9.4%	.001
Generalized anxiety disorder	3.5%	19.5%	5.4%	3.9%	.001

prior six months had made no visits to either mental health care or general medical care providers (Shapiro et al., 1984).

Together with the affective and substance abuse disorders, anxiety disorders affect large numbers of the population. Assuming the lowest ECA estimate to be true (11.1 percent for phobias, panic disorder, and obsessive-compulsive disorder for both sexes), we are concerned with 20 million people in the U.S. population. If the follow-up study of the natural history of the anxiety disorders by Wheeler et al. holds true, over 50 percent of patients will remain unimproved or disabled after twenty years if they are not treated. These figures suggest a medical and psychiatric problem of considerable size. The availability of effective treatment at present implies the need for vigorous ascertainment of those who may benefit from it and an effective way to deliver such therapy.

REFERENCES

Helzer J, Robins L, McEvory M: Post-traumatic stress disorder in the general population. *N Engl J Med* 317:1630–1634, 1987.

Meyers J, Weissman M, Tischler G, et al. Six month prevalence of psychiatric disorders in three communities. *Arch Gen Psychiatry* 41:959–967, 1984.

Noyes R, Clarkson C, Crowe R, et al: A family study of generalized anxiety disorder. *Am J Psychiatry* 144:1019–1024, 1987.

Robins L, Helzer J, Weissman M, et al: Lifetime prevalence of specific psychiatric disorders in three sites. *Arch Gen Psychiatry* 41:949–958, 1984.

Shapiro S, Skinner E, Kessler L, et al: Utilization of health and mental health services. *Arch Gen Psychiatry* 41:971–978, 1984.

Tyrer P: Classification of anxiety disorders: A critique of DSM-III. *J Affective Disord* 11:99–104, 1986.

Tyrer P, Alexander J, Remington V, et al: Relationship between neurotic symptoms and neurotic diagnosis: A longitudinal study. *J Affective Disord* 13:13–31, 1987.

Wheeler E, White P, Reed E, et al: Neurocirculatory asthenia (anxiety neurosis, effort syndrome, neurasthenia): A twenty year follow-up study of one hundred and seventy-three patients. *JAMA* 142:878–888, 1950.

Woodruff R, Murphy G, Herjanic M: The natural history of affective disorders. 1. Symptoms of 72 patients at the time of index hospital admission. *J Psychiatr Res* 5:255–263, 1967.

2

Psychological Treatment for Anxiety Disorders: Adjustment Disorder with Anxious Mood, Generalized Anxiety Disorders, Panic Disorder, Agoraphobia, and Avoidant Personality Disorder

MICHAEL GELDER

It is widely believed that all forms of psychological treatment have similar therapeutic effects and that the response to any single treatment is due mainly to nonspecific factors. In recent years, cognitive and behavioral treatments have been developed to treat the various kinds of anxiety disorder, and there is accumulating evidence that these treatments have specific effects. This chapter is concerned mainly with a review of some of these newer psychological treatments for anxiety disorders, although reference will also be made, where appropriate, to the older methods of relaxation, counseling, and dynamic psychotherapy. The treatment of four kinds of anxiety disorder will be considered: adjustment disorder with anxious mood, generalized anxiety disorders, panic disorder, agoraphobia, and avoidant personality disorder. The chapter consists of two parts. The shorter first part describes the general psychological abnormalities present in all anxiety disorders. The second part describes the specific psychological abnormalities found in the five disorders that are the subject of this chapter and discusses their psychological treatment. The treatment of the remaining anxiety disorders—posttraumatic stress disorder, simple and social phobias, and obsessive-compulsive disorder—is considered in the next chapter.

PSYCHOLOGICAL ABNORMALITIES PRESENT
IN ALL ANXIETY DISORDERS

Anxiety is a normal emotional state. Anxiety disorders differ from normal states of anxiety in being of an intensity that is out of proportion to the causes for anxiety and in being unduly prolonged. Of these two features, it is the prolongation of the mood state that is particularly characteristic of anxiety disorders. For this reason it is useful, when studying the psychopathology of specific anxiety disorders, to pay particular attention to factors that maintain the anxiety response beyond the point at which it is appropriate. Because these maintaining factors differ in the various kinds of anxiety disorder, they will be described in subsequent sections of this chapter. Here we consider the normal anxiety response and the features that the different kinds of anxiety disorder have in common.

The normal anxiety response has three principal components: physiological arousal, cognitive processes, and coping strategies. The first of these, *physiological arousal,* has three parts: autonomic arousal, increases in tension in skeletal muscles, and increased ventilation of the lungs. All three can be thought of as part of a preparation for the increased muscular activity that accompanies approach or avoidance ("fight or flight"). These features are well known and will not be discussed further here. The *cognitive processes* in normal anxiety seem to include increased attention to potentially dangerous aspects of the environment and appraisal of other information about the environment for possible threat (Butler and Mathews, 1987). The *coping strategies* include avoidance of some potentially dangerous situations and approach to others with the intention of reducing their danger. These last two components of the anxiety response require some additional comments, but it will be more convenient to make these when considering their role in anxiety disorders.

In anxiety disorders, one or more of these components of the anxiety response is abnormal. Arousal may be excessive either because the person's autonomic system is unusually responsive to stressors or because an excessively threatening appraisal is made of potential stressors. Variations in autonomic responsiveness to stressful stimuli seem to be partly under genetic control. Variations in the appraisal of information about the environment are part of the cognitive processes in anxiety disorders that will be considered next.

In anxiety disorders, cognitive processes may be distorted in several ways. First, attention is often focused on information from the person's internal environment instead of the more adaptive focus on the external environment found in normal anxiety. Thus the person with an anxiety disorder focuses more on personal thoughts and body processes than on the external world. Since these thoughts and body processes are themselves disturbed by anxiety, a vicious circle of anxiety may be set up. A second cognitive distortion is that the appraisal of the dangerousness of situations may be unrealistic, with excessive concern about possible harm in circumstances that are in fact quite safe. A third cognitive distortion is a reduced ability to reason logically about fearful thoughts, especially at times of high anxiety (Beck and Rush, 1975).

Coping strategies may be maladaptive in several ways. A common problem is excessive reliance on avoidance of anxiety situations and insufficient use of approach behavior. This pattern of behavior deprives the person of experiences that could result in deconditioning of psychophysiological responses and reappraisal of the dangerousness of situations. A second poor coping strategy consists of developing inadequate skills for dealing with everyday problems, so that stressful circumstances are unnecessarily prolonged.

Psychological treatment attempts to modify one or more of these three components of the anxiety disorders. Relaxation, meditation, and biofeedback techniques can be used to reduce arousal. Cognitive therapy or dynamic psychotherapy can be employed to modify the cognitive disorder. Behavior therapy and the teaching of coping strategies can be used to alter maladaptive coping strategies. For some disorders, attention to one of these components is sufficient, either because only this part of the anxiety response is disordered or because a change in this one component is followed by changes in the others. In other anxiety disorders, more than one treatment technique is required. Nevertheless, it is important to remember that it is not necessary to use all three techniques in every case; such a blunderbuss approach is wasteful of treatment resources and unnecessarily demanding for the patient. In the sections that follow, an account will be given of the different combinations of treatment techniques that are required to modify the specific psychopathology of each of the anxiety disorders considered in this chapter.

ADJUSTMENT DISORDER WITH ANXIOUS MOOD

This term denotes a disorder that occurs within three months of a stressful event, is insufficiently severe to meet the criteria for an anxiety disorder, and does not persist for more than six months. These disorders are frequent among anxious people who seek help from family practitioners, and many of the anxiolytic drugs prescribed are for these conditions.

In terms of the discussion in the previous section, these disorders are normal responses to stressful events or changes in the person's routine of living. The psychopathology has not been studied systematically but probably resembles that of a normal anxiety response without important maintaining factors. For this reason, treatment can be of a simple kind. An obvious form of treatment is to reduce the excessive arousal by training in relaxation, meditation, or biofeedback. However, this treatment is seldom practical because the training generally requires several weeks to produce a worthwhile effect, and patients need immediate help. For this reason, these methods of reducing arousal are discussed in the section on generalized anxiety disorders.

Counseling

The mainstay of treatment of these cases is counseling. This may be either nonspecific or directed to improving problem solving. There have been no systematic studies of counseling for adjustment disorders, but two studies at Oxford have produced relevant information. The first study concerned a group of patients with acute anxiety reactions as well as adjustment disorders. In this study (Catalan et al., 1984), nonspecific counseling techniques were used by general practitioners. The counseling was quite brief: less than ten minutes per weekly session. The benign nature of the anxiety response was explained, together with the origins and significance of the various psychological and physical symptoms experienced by the patient. Patients were helped to identify important stressful events and encouraged to consider steps to overcome them. No drugs were prescribed to patients receiving counseling. In the investigation, patients who would normally have been treated by the general practitioner with anxiolytic drugs were allocated randomly either to counseling or to treatment with these drugs. Progress was assessed in several ways. All the measures of change indicated that the patients who received counseling improved as much as those who received drugs; systematic inquiries showed that this result was not due to the greater use of unprescribed drugs or alcohol by the patients who received counseling. This finding is important, though not surprising, since most anxiety disorders of this kind treated by general practitioners improve within a few weeks. However, although about one-half of the patients improved quickly with counseling or drugs, about one-third still had anxiety symptoms six months after the start of treatment. The second study showed how these results could be improved.

Problem Solving

One reason why some patients do not recover with simple counseling might be that they are less able than others to deal with the problems that provoked the anxiety. For this reason, a second study was carried out to examine the effects of a more elaborate form of counseling for persistent cases (Catalan and Gath, 1989). This counseling was intended to improve the patients' ability to cope with stressors by teaching simple problem-solving skills. Patients were selected who resembled those with more persistent anxiety in the first study, and were allocated randomly either to this form of counseling, given by a psychiatrist, or to treatment with anxiolytic drugs by the general practitioner. The patients who received counseling improved significantly more than the others. Moreover, their state six months after the start of treatment was comparable to that of patients in the first study who recovered quickly.

These findings presumably indicate that in a minority of patients with acute stress and adjustment disorders presenting to general practitioners, symptoms are prolonged by poor coping skills, with failure to resolve stressful problems. The findings also show the value of increasing these skills. However, even with this more elaborate form of counseling, a few patients have persistent anxiety. These are the patients with generalized, panic and phobic, panic, and other anxiety disorders. Their treatment is considered in the following sections of this chapter and in the next chapter.

GENERALIZED ANXIETY DISORDERS

These disorders are more severe than the adjustment disorders and, by definition, last for more than six months. They have a more complex psychopathology than the adjustment disorders considered in the previous section. The cognitive disorder in generalized anxiety is mainly of the kind that has already been described as common to all anxiety disorders. It has four components. The first component of the disorder consists of repeated worrying thoughts about a multitude of problems, the most frequent of which are concerned with illness and dying, inability to cope, loss of control, and social embarrassment (Beck et al., 1974). The second component consists of selective attention to cues for danger found also in normal, short-lived states of anxiety together with an appraisal of circumstances as more dangerous than they really are (Butler and Mathews, 1983; Mathews and MacLeod, 1985; MacLeod et al., 1986). The third component is a general approach to life that engenders unnecessary stress—for example, excessive striving for success. The fourth component consists of poor coping behavior, especially excessive avoidance of situations that cause anxiety behaviors (Butler et al., 1987). The presence of avoidance may seem unexpected in generalized rather than phobic anxiety. However, avoidance is present, though of a different pattern, being more diffuse and often involving avoidance of internal cues, such as thinking about problems (Borkovec, 1976).

Relaxation Training and Related Methods

Several psychological treatments have been used for generalized anxiety disorders. Treatments of the first kind, intended to reduce the persistently high level of arousal, are relaxation training, meditation, and biofeedback. There are several techniques for training in relaxation, all of which derive from Jacobson's progressive relaxation (Jacobson, 1938, 1964). Although this procedure can produce satisfactory relaxation, it is so lengthy that several shorter forms have been developed, for example, by Bernstein and Borkovec (1973). Other variants of Jacobson's original technique have been designed to enable patients to relax at the times when anxiety is provoked, rather than in the intervals between episodes of anxiety. This requires the ability to relax when engaging in activities, not just when lying on a couch or sitting quietly in a chair. Such methods are called "applied relaxation," and several variants have been described (Goldfried and Trier, 1974; Sherman and Plummer, 1973; Deffenbacher and Snyder, 1976; Ost, 1988). Although good effects have been reported in the treatment of short-lived anxiety responses to public speaking and other stressful situations, traditional forms of relaxation have not been shown to be effective with generalized anxiety disorders (Le Boeuf and Lodge, 1980), though Ost's method may be more effective.

Most forms of meditation include an element of relaxation. Although yoga and transcendental meditation have been claimed to produce reductions in arousal comparable to those of relaxation training (Wallace et al., 1971), subsequent investigations have not shown substantial effects (Holmes, 1987). These methods have the advantage that many patients find them more interesting and involving than relaxation training, and therefore practice more diligently (Raskin et al., 1980; Lehrer et al., 1983).

Biofeedback of muscle (EMG) has been used as an alternative to relaxation to reduce arousal, and its effects have been shown to be similar to those of traditional relaxation training (Canter et al., 1975; Lavellée, et al. 1977; Le Boeuf and Lodge, 1980; Lehrer, 1982). Biofeedback has also been used as an adjunct to relaxation training (e.g., Townsend et al., 1975); however, the addition of feedback has not been shown to produce significant extra benefit (Raskin et al., 1980).

Cognitive Therapy

The poor results obtained with all these methods of relaxation may be explained by their failure to deal with cognitive and other maintaining factors of generalized anxiety disorders. Several forms of cognitive treatment have been used to modify the cognitions that characterize generalized anxiety disorders. Meichenbaum (1977) was one of the first to develop methods in which patients were helped to identify irrational anxiety-provoking thoughts and to replace them with rational, calming thoughts. This therapy has been used with good effect in the treatment of patients who experience anxiety when speaking in public or performing on the stage (Barrios and Shigetomi, 1979). However, when applied to generalized anxiety disorders, the results have not been impressive (Woodward and Jones, 1980).

A more elaborate cognitive treatment for generalized anxiety disorder has been suggested by Beck, who developed it from his "cognitive therapy for depression." In the first stage of this treatment, irrational anxiety-provoking thoughts are identified by interviewing patients and encouraging them to keep records of their thoughts when anxious. In the second stage, these thoughts are challenged by questioning their validity and identifying errors of logic that lie behind them. In the third stage, dysfunctional beliefs are uncovered and then undermined by repeated questioning. In the treatment of generalized anxiety disorders, Beck's cognitive therapy has been shown to have more effect than no treatment. Compared with lorazepam, cognitive therapy is slower in its action (Lindsay et al., 1987). It is not known how its effects compare with those of continuing treatment with benzodiazepines, except that cognitive therapy is, of course, free from the risk of dependence that goes with prolonged treatment with these drugs. Beck's cognitive therapy seems to produce effects similar to those of Suinn's version of "anxiety management training" (Lindsay et al., 1987); to those of behavioral treatment given with no specific attempts to elicit or modify cognitions (Durham and Turvey, 1987); and to those of nondirective counseling (Blowers et al., 1987).

Anxiety Management

None of the treatments of generalized anxiety disorder reviewed so far has been shown to have a striking therapeutic effect. Investigations of similar patients at Oxford led to the conclusion that this is because these treatments fail to deal with one of the important maintaining factors in generalized anxiety disorder: avoidance of situations that provoke anxiety. As noted earlier in this section, this avoidance is less focused than that occurring in phobic disorders, in which it is easy to identify a few avoided situations. Instead there is incomplete avoidance of a wide range of anxiety-provoking situations, some in the external environment, others internal to the patient—for example, thinking about problems. This avoidance prevents deconditioning, reappraisal of danger, and problem solving, and it is important to overcome it. The treatment developed for generalized anxiety disorder by the Oxford research group is directed to all three aspects of the psychopathology of generalized anxiety disorder: relaxation to reduce arousal; cognitive procedures to identify anxious thoughts and replace them with positive thoughts; measures to improve coping skills; and, importantly, efforts to replace avoidance of anxiety-provoking situations by approach to them. This treatment, known as "anxiety management," has been evaluated in several clinical studies. It has had a substantial therapeutic effect in generalized anxiety disorders, greater than that seen in a waiting list control group (Jannoun et al., 1982; Butler et al., 1987). Also, the preliminary results of a continuing investigation indicate that although exposure and relaxation have their own worthwhile therapeutic effects, the cognitive component is important as well (Butler et al., 1987). This combination of cognitive and behavioral techniques, which deals with the two most important maintaining factors in generalized anxiety disorders, appears to produce good results. However, a final assessment of its value will require further clinical trials in which the various psychological treatments for generalized anxiety disorder are compared with each other and with anxiolytic drug therapy over a prolonged period of follow-up.

PANIC DISORDER

Since it is widely believed that panic disorder has a biological cause and requires pharmacological treatment, it is appropriate to begin by explaining why a psychological treatment should be thought appropriate for the condition. To understand this, it is necessary to consider the way in which the psychopathology of panic attacks and panic disorder differs from that of generalized anxiety disorder.

Panic attacks can arise in two main ways: as a severe form of situational anxiety in phobic disorders, and without any external stimulus— either in phobic disorders or in panic disorder. Panic attacks arising without any external stimulus are generally assumed to arise from a biological cause, but there is strong evidence that many, perhaps most, arise from internal psychological causes. These psychological causes are of two kinds. The first is the anticipation of fear-provoking situations and of the state of anxiety that will occur in them ("fear of fear"). The second psychological cause is a more specific fear related to certain kinds of bodily sensation, notably palpitations and dizziness. This fear is of a particular kind: a fear that the bodily sensation is the immediate forerunner of a serious medical emergency such as a heart attack.

There are three main sources of evidence for these specific cognitions. First, when panic disorder patients and generalized anxiety disorder patients are questioned in the same way about their thoughts when anxious, the former report significantly more thoughts about sudden illness, loss of control, and dying (Hibbert, 1984). These thoughts usually occur immediately after the person has become aware of a somatic sensation such as palpitations. As explained above, the thoughts are concerned with some immediate physical or mental catastrophe such as a heart attack, and it is the immediacy of the person's concerns that distinguishes this thinking from the longer-term apprehensions about ill-health that characterize hypochondriacal patients. These findings have led to the suggestion that panic attacks arise when a person has an enduring tendency to interpret sensations from the body in a catastrophic way—for example, to interpret palpitations as evidence of an impending heart attack (Clark, 1986; Clark et al., 1988). It is also suggested that such misinterpretation leads to an increasing spiral of anxiety, with sensations such as palpitations leading to anxiety, which in turn leads to an increase in palpitations.

The second piece of evidence about the cognitive abnormality in panic disorder has been obtained in a contextual priming experiment (Clark et al., 1988). Contextual priming tasks make use of the everyday observation that when asked to read words aloud, a person will respond more quickly to a word that is expected than to a word that is unexpected. In the particular contextual priming task used to demonstrate the cognitions associated with panic attacks, subjects were shown an incomplete sentence (for example, "If I had palpitations, I could be . . .") followed by a word to be read aloud. This word was chosen from one of two lists, each of which contained words that could complete the sentence. Words in the two lists were matched for frequency of occurrence in the English language. The first kind of word was related to the hypothesized concerns of panic disorder patients (for example, "dying"); the second kind of word was unrelated to these concerns (for example, "excited"). After reading the incomplete sentence, patients with panic disorder were found to respond significantly more quickly to words of the first kind than to words of the second kind. Controls responded at the same speed to both kinds of word. When the same words were shown without the incomplete sentence, panic disorder patients responded to the two kinds of word at the same speed, indicating that they did not have a general tendency to respond more quickly to the first kind of word. These findings strongly suggest that panic disorder patients expect physical symptoms to be followed by immediate and serious illness in a way that other people do not.

The third piece of evidence for the existence of specific cognitions in panic disorder is from an experiment designed to activate the cognitions (Ehlers et al., 1988). Two kinds of heart rate feedback were presented to panic disorder patients and to normal subjects: accurate feedback and feedback indicating a heart rate faster than the true heart rate. Panic disorder patients were made substantially more anxious by the false than by the true feedback, but normal controls became only a little more anxious. Similar results have been reported by Clark et al. (1988). These findings can be explained if the link between awareness of heart action and anxiety is made by "catastrophic" cognitions linking rapid heartbeat to a heart attack or another impending medial emergency.

Relaxation Training

Several kinds of psychological treatment have been used for panic disorder. The simplest is "applied relaxation," which has been used to reduce arousal and thereby enable patients to control panic attacks (Ost, 1988). With panic disorder patients, applied relaxation has been shown to be more effective than "progressive relaxation," used between attacks. These findings are of considerable interest, since traditional methods of relaxation should not have any direct effect on the specific cognitions identified by Clark. Ost's method differs in the rationale given for treatment, which stresses the importance of a vicious circle of worry and increasing tension. It is possible, therefore, that it may have an indirect effect on cognitions.

Cognitive Therapy

Clark and his colleagues (Clark et al., 1985; Salkovskis et al., 1986) have developed a special kind of cognitive therapy designed to alter the catastrophic cognitions that characterize panic disorder. The first step in treatment is to reproduce the feared symptoms in a safe way. This is usually done with voluntary hyperventilation, which regularly evokes palpitations, dizziness, and other relevant symptoms. The appearance of the feared symptoms in this way provokes the catastrophic cognitions, and this sequence is pointed out to the patient, who is encouraged to consider whether the bodily symptoms that occur at the beginning of the "spontaneous" attacks of panic are caused by hyperventilation or in some equally benign way. Subsequently, the cognitions are undermined further by questioning their logical basis and by arranging "behavioral experiments" to test their validity. These procedures are usually followed by a rapid and substantial reduction in the frequency of panic attacks; this improvement has been found to be maintained two years after treatment (Clark et al., 1985; Salkovskis et al., 1986).

Other Psychological Treatments

Applied relaxation and Clark's special kind of cognitive therapy are not the only psychological treatments for panic disorder. Good results have been reported with the use of anxiety management (Gitlin et al., 1988). Barlow (1988) has developed a method, combining cognitive and behavioral techniques, in which the central feature is repeated exposure to the sensations that provoke anxiety. Results similar to those of Clark et al. have been reported.

Until these various methods have been compared with one another in randomized clinical trials, it cannot be determined which is most effective; at present, the evidence favors applied relaxation and the form of cognitive therapy developed by Clark. Whichever of these methods emerges as the most successful, it is clear that panic disorder responds to psychological as well as pharmacological treatment.

AGORAPHOBIA

The most obvious features of the psychopathology of agoraphobia are those mentioned already: high arousal, avoidance behavior, and anticipatory anxiety. Many agoraphobic patients have spontaneous panic attacks. These patients seem to have the tendency to make catastrophic misinterpretations about bodily symptoms described in the section on panic disorder. Finally, it has been suggested that the condition is often maintained by secondary gain and by stressful family problems.

There is an increasingly popular belief that most cases of agoraphobia arise from panic disorder. According to this belief, the primary changes are panic attacks and situational anxiety, anticipatory anxiety, and avoidance behavior are secondary features arising from conditioning and cognitive learning. If this view is correct, treatment directed to these secondary features should reduce them but should have little effect on the panic attacks (Klein et al., 1987). This is the rationale for drug treatment, used to control the panic disorder underlying panic disorder, and its combination with exposure treatment, used to reduce the secondary features. The alternative view is that all aspects of agoraphobia, including any spontaneous panics, have psychological causes. If this is correct, the whole treatment can be psychological, without any need to use drugs.

Relaxation and Problem Solving

The different kinds of psychological treatment for agoraphobia have different aspects of the psychopathology as their targets. Applied relaxation has been used to reduce the state of high arousal provoked by phobic stimuli. Good results have been reported by Ost et al. (1984), although the findings have not yet been confirmed by others. Problem-solving techniques have been used to reduce the stressful results of family and other problems, but their effect is small and is significantly less than that of behavioral treatment, which will be described next (Cullington et al., 1984).

Exposure Treatment

The most frequently used treatment for agoraphobia is directed to the most prominent aspect of the psychopathology—the avoidance behavior. This treatment, usually called "exposure," encourages repeated approaches to any anxiety-provoking situations that have been persistently avoided. Exposure can be carried out in several ways, all of which produce substantial improvement in agoraphobia (see Marks, 1987, for a review and Trull et al., 1988, for the results of a meta-analysis). The variations in the basic method are as follows: Exposure can be carried out rapidly with high anxiety (a procedure known as "flooding"), or slowly with minimal anxiety ("desensitization"); and by returning to actual situations that have been avoided ("exposure in practice"), or by imagining a return to these situations ("exposure in imagination"). Evidence shows that exposure in practice is more effective than exposure in imagination, and that exposure at an intermediate level of anxiety is as effective as exposure at a very high or a very low level (Marks, 1987).

Several other variants of exposure treatment have been advocated. Patients can practice alone, with the therapist, or with another person—usually the spouse or a close friend. Practice with the therapist does not seem to confer any substantial advantage over practice alone (Ghosh et al., 1987; Mitchelson et al., 1988), at least for patients who are willing to practice on their own, possibly because it fails to develop patients' confidence in their ability to help themselves. The involvement of the spouse can help to motivate the patient and can create a more cooperative relationship between the marriage partners, but it is not certain whether it leads to more improvement than an equal amount of unaccompanied practice. Cobb et al. (1984) found that it did not have this effect, while Barlow et al. (1984) found that it did.

The belief that agoraphobia is a secondary sequence of panic disorder has led to treatment in which a drug (usually imipramine) is combined with exposure treatment. Opinions differ about the value of this combination. In one study, no increased benefit was found with the addition of imipramine to exposure for a group of agoraphobics who were free from depressive disorder (Marks et al., 1983; Cohen et al., 1984). In other studies, also of agoraphobics without definite evidence of a depressive disorder, the combined treatment has been found to be more effective than exposure without drugs (Mavissakalian et al., 1983; Telch et al., 1985).

Cognitive Therapy

Several attempts have been made to treat agoraphobia with cognitive therapy. The aims of this treatment differed in different studies, being directed to various aspects of the cognitive disorder. A standard form of cognitive therapy intended to change anticipatory and situational anxiety was found to be no more effective, and probably less so, than exposure (Emmelkamp et al., 1978, 1986; Emmelkamp and Mersch, 1982). Better results were reported when cognitive therapy procedures was combined with exposure treatment. The cognitive therapy was usually directed to anticipatory anxiety. This symptom can be modified by explaining how it has arisen and how it can exacerbate the other symptoms; and by teaching simple ways of coping with panic attacks, using relaxation and distraction, and repeating reassuring phrases to counteract anxious thoughts. This combination of exposure and cognitive therapy has been shown to have a greater therapeutic effect than exposure alone (Marchione et al., 1987).

Cognitive Behavioral Treatment

The group at Oxford has developed a special form of treatment for agoraphobia that combines exposure and cognitive procedures, and includes measures to reduce dependency and increase motivation. Daily exposure is carried out from home, rather than from the psychiatric clinic, with help from another person, usually the patient's spouse. Information is given about the nature of panic attacks, with instruction in ways of overcoming the anxiety by using applied relaxation, distraction, and substitution of reassuring thoughts for anxiety-evoking cognitions. Written information and instructions are provided for the patient and the helper, so that both will have a clear understanding of the principles and practice of treatment and will thereby be more able to deal with unexpected circumstances. This treatment, sometimes known as "programmed practice," has been shown to be more effective than control treatments (Mathews et al., 1977; Jannoun et al., 1980).

Exposure treatment for agoraphobia has been studied by many investigators. An overall view of the results has been obtained by Jacobson et al. (1988), who reanalyzed data from 11 studies. They found an average improvement rate of 58 percent at the end of treatment and of 60 percent at follow-up. However, the average of recovery (rather than improvement) rate was only 27 percent at the end of treatment and 34 percent at follow-up. These were overall results from all forms of exposure treatment. The authors' independent reanalysis of the Oxford trial of programmed practice showed strikingly better results, with 82 percent improvement at the end of treatment and 93 percent at follow-up, as well as 46 percent recovery at the end of treatment and 57 percent at follow-up. However, while these figures show the value of this combination of practice at home, training in panic management, involvement of the spouse, and written instructions, the recovery rate is still less than 60 percent.

Follow-up studies with all kinds of exposure treatment indicate that the improvement reached at the end of treatment continues in the group for up to four years (Marks, 1971; Emmelkamp and Kuipers, 1979; McPherson et al., 1980; Munby and Johnston, 1980; Burns et al., 1986; Lelliott et al., 1987). However, this overall result hides the fact that some patients go on improving, while a few relapse. The obvious next step is to use the cognitive treatment for panic disorder, described in the previous section, and determine whether this improves the long-term results obtained with the other kinds of cognitive behavior treatment, in which the cognitive procedures are directed to the more general issue of fear of fear. Only preliminary data are available on the effects of cognitive therapy for panic in agoraphobia. These indicate that such treatment can reduce substantially the frequency of panic attacks in agoraphobia. In the study of Clark et al. (1984), the frequency fell from 10 to 2 per week, and this improvement was maintained at follow-up two years later. Clearly, further studies are needed before advice can be given about the best form of cognitive therapy to combine with exposure treatment for agoraphobia.

AVOIDANT PERSONALITY DISORDER

Patients with this disorder have an enduring tendency to become anxious and to avoid stressful situations, a tendency that begins in adolescence. In contrast to the other disorders considered in this chapter, there have been no clinical trials of psychological treatment directed specifically to this disorder. For this reason, opinions must be based on clinical experience.

Dynamic Psychotherapy

The usual treatment for avoidant personality disorder is dynamic psychotherapy. In this treatment, attention is directed to ways of thinking that result in anxiety in situations that other people do not find threatening. Unlike cognitive therapy, the aim is to explore the origins of the ways of thinking in past experience and, by making the patient aware of this development, to help him or her think in more adaptive ways. This awareness may be increased by interpretations linking past experience with present ideas and behavior, or by symbolic interpretations. Particular attention is paid to thoughts and feelings that are denied or disowned, as they appear reflected in relationships outside treatment or in the transference. In considering current problems, attention is directed to conflicts among relationships, wishes, and values.

Cognitive Therapy

The essential features of avoidant personality disorder include fear of criticism by others, timidity, avoidance of social and occupational situations, awkwardness in company, and a tendency to avoid stressful situations. Some of these problems can be treated with cognitive-behavioral methods similar to those used for social phobia (described in the next chapter). However, the underlying lack of self-confidence and the overcautious approach to activities sometimes make this approach difficult because it requires the patient to test new ways of behaving in everyday situations. When these features of the disorder are marked, clinical experience indicates that treatment with dynamic psychotherapy is more likely to be helpful.

CONCLUSION

When psychological treatment is directed to the specific psychopathology of the anxiety disorders considered in this chapter, good results can be obtained. Although some of the treatments take more time than the prescription of drugs, this extra time is justified because the problem of dependence on anxiolytic drugs is avoided and patients acquire coping skills that can be employed at future times of stress. This possibility of secondary prevention is one of the most attractive features of these psychological treatments for anxiety disorders.

REFERENCES

Barlow DH: *Anxiety and Its Disorders: The Nature and Treatment of Anxiety and Panic*. New York, Guilford Press.
Barlow DH, O'Brien GT, Last CG: Couples treatment of agoraphobia. *Behav Ther* 15:41–58, 1984.

Barrios BA, Shigetomi CC: Coping-skills training for the management of anxiety: A critical review. *Behav Ther* 10:491–522, 1979.

Beck AT, Laude R, Bohnert M: Ideational components of anxiety neurosis. *Arch Gen Psychiatry* 31:319–325, 1974.

Beck AT, Rush AJ: A cognitive model of anxiety formation and anxiety resolution, in Sarason ID, Spielberger CD (eds): *Stress and Anxiety*. Washington, Hemisphere Publishing, 1975, pp 69–80.

Bernstein DA, Borkovec TD: *Progressive Relaxation Training*. Champaign, IL, Research Press, 1973.

Blowers C, Cobb J, Mathews A: Generalized anxiety—a controlled treatment study. *Behav Res Ther* 25:493–502, 1987.

Borkovec TD: Physiological and cognitive processes in the regulation of anxiety, in Schivarty GE, Shapiro D (eds): *Consciousness and Self-Regulation: Advances of Research,* Vol I. New York, Plenum Press, 1976, pp 261–312.

Borkovec TD, Mathews A: Treatment of nonphobic anxiety disorders: A comparison of non-directive, cognitive, and coping desensitization therapy. *J Consult Clin Psychol* 56:877–844, 1988.

Borkovec TD, Mathews A, Chambers A, et al: The effects of relaxation training with cognitive or non-directive therapy and the role of relaxation induced anxiety in the treatment of generalized anxiety. *J Consult Clin Psychol* 55:883–888, 1987.

Burns LE, Thorpe GL, Cavallaro LA: Agoraphobia eight years after behavioural treatment: A follow-up study with interview, self-report and behavioural data. *Behav Ther* 17:580–591, 1986.

Butler G, Gelder M, Hibbert G, et al: Anxiety management—developing effective strategies. *Behav Res Ther* 25:517–522, 1987.

Butler G, Mathews A: Cognitive processes in anxiety. *Adv Behav Res Ther* 5:51–62, 1983.

Butler G, Mathews A: Anticipatory anxiety and risk perception. *Cogn Ther Res* 11:551–565, 1987.

Canter A, Kondo CY, Knott JRA: A comparison of EMG biofeedback and progressive muscle relaxation training with anxiety neurotics. *Br J Psychiatry* 127:470–477, 1975.

Catalan J, Gath D: A problem-solving approach in the treatment of emotional problems in primary care: A controlled clinical trial. Submitted for publication.

Catalan J, Gath D, Edmonds G, et al: The effects of non-prescribing of anxiolytics in general practice: I. Controlled evaluation. *Br J Psychiatry* 144:593–602, 1984.

Clark DM: A cognitive approach to panic. *Behav Res Ther* 23:585–600, 1986.

Clark DM, Salkovskis PM, Chalkley AJ: Respiratory control as a treatment for panic attacks. *J Behav Ther Exp Psychiatry* 16:23–30, 1985.

Clark DM, Salkovskis PM, Gelder MG, et al: Tests of a cognitive theory of panic, in Hand I, Wittchen HV (eds): *Panic and Phobias,* Vol. 2. Berlin, Springer-Verlag, 1988, pp 41–53.

Cobb JP, Mathews AM, Childs-Clarke A, et al: The spouse as co-therapist in the treatment of agoraphobia. *Br J Psychiatry* 144:282–287, 1984.

Cohen SD, Monteiro W, Marks IM: Two-year follow-up of agoraphobics after exposure and imipramine. *Br J Psychiatry* 144:276–281, 1984.

Cullington A, Butler G, Hibbert G, et al: Problem-solving: Not a treatment for agoraphobia. *Behav Ther* 15:280–286, 1984.

Deffenbacher JL, Snyder AL: Relaxation as self-control in the treatment of test and other anxieties. *Psychol Rep* 39:379–385, 1976.

Durham RC, Turvey AA: Cognitive therapy vs. behaviour therapy in the treatment of chronic general anxiety. *Behav Res Ther* 25:229–234, 1987.

Ehlers A, Margraf J, Roth WT, et al: Anxiety induced by false heart rate feedback in patients with panic disorder. *Behav Res Ther* 21:1–11, 1988.

Emmelkamp PMG, Brilman E, Kuiper H, et al: The treatment of agoraphobia: A comparison of self-instructional training, rational emotive therapy, and exposure in vivo. *Behav Modification* 10:37–53, 1986.

Emmelkamp PMG, Kuipers ACM: Agoraphobia: A follow up study four years after treatment. *Br J Psychiatry* 134:352–355, 1979.

Emmelkamp PMG, Kuipers CM, Eggeraat JB: Cognitive modification versus prolonged exposure in vivo: A comparison with agoraphobics as subjects. *Behav Res Ther* 16:33–41, 1978.

Emmelkamp PMG, Mersch PP: Cognition and exposure in vivo in the treatment of agoraphobia: Short-term and delayed effects. *Cogn Ther Res* 6:77–86, 1982.

Frank JD: *Persuasion and Healing: A Comparative Study of Psychotherapy.* Baltimore, Johns Hopkins University Press, 1961.

Frank JD: The psychotherapy of anxiety, in Grinspoon L (ed.): *Psychiatry Update: The American Psychiatric Association Annual Review.* Washington, DC, American Psychiatric Press, 1984, pp 418–426.

Ghosh A, Marks IM, Plienis AJ, et al: Self treatment of agoraphobia by exposure. *Behav Ther* 18:3–16, 1987.

Gitlin B, Martin J, Shear MK, et al: Behaviour therapy for panic disorder. *J Nerv Ment Dis* 173:742–743, 1988.

Goldfried MR, Trier CS: Effectiveness of relaxation as an active coping skill. *J Abnorm Psychol* 83:348–355, 1974.

Hibbert GA: Ideational components of anxiety: Their origin and content. *Br J Psychiatry* 144:618–624, 1984.

Holmes DS: The influence of meditation versus rest on physiological arousal: A second examination, in West MA (ed): *The Psychology of Meditation.* Oxford, Clarendon Press, 1987, pp 81–103.

Jacobson E: *Progressive Relaxation.* Chicago, University of Chicago Press, 1938.

Jacobson E: *Anxiety and Tension Control.* Philadelphia, JB Lippincott, 1964.

Jacobson NS, Wilson L, Tupper C: The clinical significance of treatment gains resulting from exposure-based interventions for agoraphobia. *Behav Ther* 19:539–554, 1988.

Jannoun L, Munby M, Catalan J, et al: A home-based treatment program for agoraphobia: Replication and controlled evaluation. *Behav Ther* 11:294–305, 1980.

Jannoun L, Oppenheimer C, Gelder MG: A self-help treatment programme for anxiety state patients. *Behav Ther* 13:103–111, 1982.

Klein DF, Ross DC, Cohen P: Panic and avoidance in agoraphobia: Application of path analysis to treatment studies. *Arch Gen Psychiatry* 44:377–385, 1987.

Lavellée Y, Lamontagne Y, Pinard G, et al: Effects of EMG biofeedback, diazepam, and their combination on chronic anxiety. *J Psychosom Res* 21:65–71, 1977.

Le Boeuf A, Lodge JA: A comparison of frontalis EMG feedback training and progressive relaxation in the treatment of chronic anxiety. *Br J Psychiatry* 137:279–284, 1980.

Lehrer P: Psychophysiological effects of progressive relaxation in anxiety neurotic patients and of progressive relaxation and alpha feedback in non-patients. *J Consult Clin Psychol* 46:389–404, 1978.

Lehrer PM: How to relax and not to relax: A re-evaluation of the work of Edmund Jacobson. *Behav Res Ther* 20:417–428, 1982.

Lehrer P, Woolfolk RL, Rooney AJ, et al: Progressive relaxation and meditation: A study of psychophysiological and therapeutic differences between two techniques. *Behav Res Ther* 21:651–662, 1983.

Lelliott PT, Marks IM, Monteiro WO, et al: Agoraphobics 5 years after imipramine and exposure, outcome and predictors. *J Nervous Ment Dis* 175:599–605, 1987.

Lindsay WR, Gamsu CV, McLaughlin E, et al: A controlled trial of treatments for generalized anxiety. *Br J Clin Psychol* 26:3–15, 1987.

MacLeod C, Mathews A, Tata P: Attentional bias in emotional disorders. *J Abnorm Psychol* 95:15–20, 1986.

Marchione KE, Michelson L, Greenwald M, et al: Cognitive behavioural treatment of agoraphobia. *Behav Res Ther* 25:319–328, 1987.

Marks IM: Phobic disorders four years after treatment, a prospective follow up. *Br J Psychiatry* 118:683–688, 1971.

Marks IM: *Fears, Phobias, and Rituals.* New York, Oxford University Press, 1987.

Marks IM, Gray S, Cohen D, et al: Imipramine and brief therapist-aided exposure in agoraphobics having self-exposure homework. *Arch Gen Psychiatry* 40:153–162, 1983.

Mathews A, MacLeod C: Selective processing of threat cues in anxiety states. *Behav Res Ther* 23:563–569, 1985.

Mathews A, Teasdale J, Munby M, et al: A home-based treatment programme for agoraphobia. *Behav Ther* 8:915–924, 1977.

Mavissakalian M, Michelson L, Dealy RS: Pharmacological treatment of agoraphobia: Imipramine versus imipramine with programmed practice. *Br J Psychiatry* 143:348–355, 1983.

McPherson FM, Broughman L, McLaren L: Maintenance of improvements in agoraphobic patients treated by behavioural methods in a four-year follow-up. *Behav Res Ther* 18:150–152, 1980.

Meichenbaum D: *Cognitive Behavior Modification.* New York: Plenum Press, 1977.

Mitchelson L, Mavissakalian M, Marchione K: Cognitive, behavioural, and psychophysiological treatments of agoraphobia: a comparative outcome investigation. *Behav Ther* 19:97–120, 1988.

Munby M, Johnston DW: Agoraphobia: The long term follow-up of behavioural treatment. *Br J Psychiatry* 137:418–427, 1980.

Ost LG: Applied relaxation vs. progressive relaxation in the treatment of panic disorder. *Behav Res Ther* 26:13–33, 1988.

Ost LG: Behaviour therapy in generalized anxiety disorder: an evaluative review. *Clin Psychol Rev* in press.

Ost LG, Jerremalm A, Jansson L: Individual response patterns and the effects of different behavioural methods in the treatment of agoraphobia. *Behav Res Ther* 22:697–707, 1984.

Rapee RM: Distinctions between panic disorder and generalized anxiety disorder. Clinical presentation. *Aust NZ J Psychiatry* 19:227–232, 1985.

Raskin M, Bali L, Peeke H: Muscle biofeedback and transcendental meditation. A controlled evaluation of efficacy in the treatment of chronic anxiety. *Arch Gen Psychiatry* 37:93–97, 1980.

Salkovskis PM, Jones DRO, Clark DM: Respiratory control in the treatment of panic attacks: Replication and extension. *Br J Psychiatry* 148:526–532, 1986.

Sherman AR, Plummer IL: Training in relaxation as a behavioural self-management skill: An exploratory investigation. *Behav Ther* 4:543–550, 1973.

Suinn RM, Richardson FC: Anxiety management training: A non-specific behaviour therapy program for anxiety control. *Behav Ther* 2:498–510, 1971.

Telch MJ, Agras WB, Roth WT, et al: Combined pharmacological and behavioural treatment for agoraphobia. *Behav Res Ther* 23:325–335, 1985.

Townsend RE, House J, Addario D: A comparison of biofeedback mediated relaxation and group therapy in the treatment of chronic anxiety. *Am J Psychiatry* 132:598–601, 1975.

Trull TJ, Nietzel MT, Main A: The use of meta-analysis to assess the clinical significance of behaviour therapy for agoraphobia. *Behav Ther* 19:527–538, 1988.

Wallace RK, Benson H, Wilson AF: A wakeful hypometabolic physiological state. *J Physiol* 221:795–799, 1971.

Woodward R, Jones RB: Cognitive restructuring treatment: A controlled trial with anxious patients. *Behav Res Ther* 18:401–407, 1980.

3

Psychosocial Treatment for Simple Phobia, Obsessive-Compulsive Disorder, Post-Traumatic Stress Disorder, and Social Phobia

WAYNE A. BOWERS

Research consistently shows that behavioral interventions are highly effective for simple phobias, agoraphobia, and obsessive-compulsive disorders (Barlow and Beck, 1984). Building on extensive earlier work, (Ellis, 1962; Beck, 1976; Meichenbaum, 1977), investigators are now studying the cognitive processes in anxiety disorders, especially nonphobic states (Clark and Beck, 1988). This has led to greater knowledge of the nature, etiology, and treatment of anxiety disorders (Beck et al., 1985; Barlow, 1988), as well as to specialized treatment manuals for panic disorder and agoraphobia (Mathews et al., 1981; Barlow and Cerny, 1988).

The most important aspect of psychosocial treatment for anxiety is exposure (Barlow, 1988). This has been shown specifically for agoraphobia (Mathews et al., 1981), panic disorder (Barlow and Cerny, 1988; Clark and Beck, 1988), generalized anxiety disorder (Deffenbacher and Suinn, 1987), simple phobia (Last, 1987), social phobia (Heimberg et al., 1987), obsessive-compulsive disorder (Steketee and Foa, 1985), and post-traumatic stress disorder (Foy et al., 1987). There are nevertheless several other components common to the psychosocial treatment of anxiety. This chapter will review these various aspects as they apply to simple phobia, obsessive-compulsive disorder, post-traumatic stress disorder, and social phobia. This review will consider only articles with true patient populations and well-defined diagnostic criteria and will be used to build a general model for the psychosocial treatment of anxiety.

SIMPLE PHOBIA

Behavioral Treatment

Systematic desensitization has been the most extensively researched behavioral approach to simple phobia (Marshall and Segal, 1988). This technique pairs relaxation with systematically introduced, anxiety-provoking images or real-life situations arranged in a graded hierarchy. There does not seem to be a clear advantage to in vivo exposure over imaginal exposure. Either format of desensitization is very effective in treating simple phobia (Mavissakalian and Barlow, 1981).

A second behavioral approach to simple phobia is modeling, which requires the patient to observe an individual effectively approach feared situations. An extension of this procedure, participant modeling, has been found to be more effective. A therapist first models nonanxious behavior in the anxiety-provoking situation, followed by the patient imitating the therapist's behavior. Research on these two approaches indicates that participant modeling is more effective with simple phobia (Bourque and Ladouceur, 1980).

A third behavioral approach is flooding, in which patients are brought in contact with one of their most feared situations, either in vivo or by imagery. Research has shown that contact in vivo is more effective than imagery (Emmelkamp, 1982). In the optimal procedure, the patient is exposed to the feared situation until anxiety has dissipated (Marshall and Segal, 1988). In addition, coping procedures may be practiced in anxiety-free situations; this, along with exposure, has been shown to be more effective than exposure alone in treating simple phobia (Williams et al., 1985). Linden (1981), however, suggests that there may be no real advantage for one type of exposure over another in the treatment of simple phobia.

Cognitive-Behavioral Treatment

As described, behavioral interventions (primarily participant modeling and exposure in vivo) are the treatments of choice in simple phobia (Emmelkamp, 1986; Marshall and Segal, 1988). However, as a result of "this unanimity of opinion, the treatment of simple phobia has been remarkably understudied" (Barlow, 1988, pp. 484–485). This lack of research has led to some confusion as to the benefit of nonexposure methods in the treatment of simple phobias.

Hayes et al. (1983) used positive self-statements designed to enhance coping with fear, in addition to desensitization, and concluded that they decreased anxiety during treatment and generated greater gains after treatment as well. Training individuals in specific behaviors to handle fearful situations also has been more effective than exposure alone with simple phobia (Williams et al., 1984, 1985). Two studies tested the use of cognitive interventions with simple phobias (Biran and Wilson, 1981; Ladouceur, 1983). Biran and Wilson compared in vivo exposure (modeling) and cognitive restructuring in individuals afraid of heights, elevators, or darkness. Those in the exposure group had significantly better scores on self-report, behavioral, and physiological measures of phobia than did those in the cognitive restructuring group.

Investigating the assumption that cognitive treatment plus participant modeling would produce the greatest, most rapid, and longest-lasting effects in the treatment of simple phobia, Ladouceur (1983) assigned individuals with dog and cat phobias to three cognitive treatment groups and a placebo control group. He found that all groups had rapid reduction of fears and significant improvement at posttest.

Because little research has been done on clinical populations, it is difficult to understand fully the role of cognitive interventions in simple phobias. Two studies on cognitive interventions suggest that these procedures may enhance treatment effectiveness when compared to strictly behavioral techniques. However, research using more complex forms of cognitive therapy and replication of current studies are needed before cognitive interventions can be recommended as a primary treatment of simple phobia.

OBSESSIVE-COMPLUSIVE DISORDER

Behavioral Treatment

As with simple phobias, exposure procedures form the basis for psychosocial treatment of obsessive-compulsive disorder (OCD). However, use of interventions such as systematic desensitization in OCD has generally been ineffective (Barlow, 1988).

Aversive techniques have been studied as treatments for OCD on the premise that an aversive event following an obsession or compulsion will suppress the behavior. These aversive methods include electric shock (Solyom and Kingstone, 1973; Kenny et al., 1978), covert desensitization, and thought stopping.

Although early research suggested otherwise, thought stopping has not proven very effective over time (Steketee and Foa, 1985). During this treatment, the patient is instructed to concentrate on the anxiety-provoking thoughts; after a short period of time, the therapist suddenly says "Stop" or uses a loud noise to disrupt the thought. After this procedure has been repeated several times and there is a reported decrease in obsessive thoughts, the control is shifted to the patient. The patient is asked to use a subvocal "Stop" when the unwanted thought occurs. Mentally seeing a stop sign or snapping a rubber band are variations on thought stopping.

A breakthrough for treating OCD occurred when Meyer (1966) showed that preventing the patient from following through with rituals while exposed to the feared object reduced overall fear and anxiety. Foa and her colleagues in Philadelphia (Steketee and Foa, 1985), as well as Rachman and Marks in England (Rachman and Hodgson, 1980), have further developed this approach.

The exposure aspect of treatment consists of bringing the patient in contact with the feared object or situation for long periods of time. This is accomplished in a graded fashion, moving from less to more intense situations. Exposure can last for periods ranging from forty-five minutes to two hours, with sessions being held up to 20 times per day. The response prevention aspect of treatment requires that the patient not engage in rituals regardless of the intensity of the discomfort. If necessary, the patient is assisted in avoiding the ritualistic behavior. (For a detailed account of this treatment, see Steketee and Foa, 1985.)

A review of the vast amount of literature on the treatment of OCD is beyond the scope of this chapter (Emmelkamp, 1986). However, several general conclusions have been drawn about behavioral treatment. Emmelkamp (1986), in his review, states that (1) gradual exposure in vivo is just as effective as flooding in vivo; (2) modeling does not seem to enhance treatment effectiveness; (3) treatment can be administered by the patient in his or her natural environment; (4) prolonged exposure is superior to shorter exposure; (5) both exposure to the distressing stimuli and response prevention of the ritual are essential to effective treatment; and (6) it may be necessary to address issues other than the obsessive-compulsive problem. Unfortunately, studies show that behavioral interventions work better with compulsions than with obsessions. Further research is needed to assess what aspects of treatment could prove effective with primarily obsessive material.

Emmelkamp (1982) reviewed the literature with long-term follow-up and suggested that treatment with behavioral therapy has a 70 percent response rate, with gains maintained for up to four and one-half years. Foa et al. (1983) followed 50 patients treated with response prevention and found that 58 percent were "much improved," 38 percent were "improved," and 4 percent were failures, according to independent judges. After three years of follow-up, 59 percent remained much improved and 17 percent were still improved, but 24 percent of this group were considered treatment failures. Foa et al. (1985) reviewed 18 controlled studies of response prevention with exposure and concluded that only 10 percent of the patients were treatment failures. Fifty-one percent of the patients in this review were symptom free or much improved, and 39 percent were improved at the completion of treatment.

Identification of variables predicting the outcome was suggested in this same study (Foa et al., 1985). Those patients who were most improved at follow-up tended to have lower levels of depression and anxiety at the start of treatment, as well as being less concerned about exposure to frightening situations.

Cognitive-Behavioral Therapy

Cognitive interventions in OCD have been less well studied in the treatment of OCD. Emmelkamp et al. (1980) determined that modifying cognitions did not enhance the effectiveness of exposure in vivo. In a subsequent study, however, Emmelkamp et al. (1988) found the rational disputation of irrational beliefs (using rational-emotive therapy) beneficial for OCD patients. In fact, cognitive interventions seemed as effective as self-controlled exposure in vivo. This is the only controlled study showing that cognitive therapy can be as effective as exposure in treating OCD; the need for replication is clear.

POST-TRAUMATIC STRESS DISORDER

Of all the anxiety disorders described in DSM III-R, post-traumatic stress disorder (PTSD) is the only one that has a clearly identifiable onset (Barlow, 1988). However, this has not led to an equally clearly identifiable treatment. Although many variations of PTSD have been described, it was not officially recognized as a separate anxiety disorder until the publication of DSM III-R (American Psychiatric Association, 1987) and whether it truly is a separate anxiety disorder is still debatable (Barlow, 1988).

The failure to conclude that PTSD is a distinct disorder has slowed research on treatment, and much of what is known comes from case studies. As in other anxiety disorders, though, exposure plays an important role in treatment. This can be imaginal exposure (Keane and Kaloupek, 1982) or in vivo. Kipper (1977) described desensitization of Israeli soldiers to traumatic memories of combat experience during the Yom Kippur War, and Kuch et al. (1984) successfully treated 30 patients with imaginal exposure after traffic accidents. Solomon and Benbenishty (1986) noted that treatment as soon as possible after the traumatic incident was very beneficial to soldiers.

Using imaginal flooding, Black and Keane (1982) treated a war veteran who had been fearful for thirty-six years. In three one-hour sessions of combat-related scenes they were able to reduce anxiety, and improvement was maintained at two-year follow-up. Similarly, Fairbank et al. (1983) used imaginal flooding with a Vietnam veteran who was almost killed and was forced to watch the torture, death, and mutilation of a fellow soldier. In this case, flooding was coupled with relaxation prior to a sixty- to seventy-minute exposure session. At six-month follow-up, the therapeutic gains were maintained.

In what Barlow (1988) suggests is the best study of PTSD, Saigh (1987) treated three Lebanese children with PTSD. Treatment involved up to sixty minutes of imaginal exposure to various trauma-related scenes in chronological order. By the end of treatment the children's fear was erased, intrusive thoughts were eliminated, and there was significant improvement in other areas, such as school performance.

What seems to be important in the treatment of other anxiety disorders is also important in the treatment of PTSD. First, there must be exposure to the feared situation (either imaginal or in vivo). Second, there must be some type of reexperiencing of the traumatic event. This aspect of the treatment must occur in an atmosphere of strong social support that will help the individual experience emotional control. Also, the individual must be offered help in redirecting attention or integrating feelings.

SOCIAL PHOBIA

Behavior Therapy

As with PTSD, social phobia disorders have received little attention from researchers (Liebowitz et al., 1985; Marshall and Segal, 1988). Treatment of social phobia can be divided into skills training and anxiety management (desensitization or flooding), with exposure as the basic component of treatment. Both types of treatment appear to be effective for socially phobic or skill deficit individuals (Biran et al., 1981; Vermilyea et al., 1984). However, earlier research on social phobia lacked adequate screening of socially phobic versus avoidant individuals, and this has led to concern over the generalizability of the findings.

More recent research has used well-defined diagnostic groups and target problems (social phobic vs. social deficits) and has shown that individuals with social deficits benefit more from skills training, while patients with phobic behavior benefit more from anxiety management, (Trower et al., 1978; Ost et al., 1981). Anxiety over speaking or writing in public apparently responds best to a combination of skills training and anxiety management (Marshall and Segal, 1988).

Cognitive-Behavioral Therapy

Cognitive restructuring has recently been coupled with exposure to treat social phobia (Heimberg et al., 1987). Two controlled outcome studies have used well-defined diagnostic criteria and detailed treatments (Butler et al., 1984; Heimberg et al., 1988). Butler et al. (1984) treated 45 patients divided into three equal groups. The first group received exposure-based exercises, the second received anxiety management (exposure with distraction techniques, cognitive restructuring, and relaxation), and the third was a waiting-list control group. The two active groups were less symptomatic than the waiting-list group at the end of treatment, and at six-month follow-up the anxiety management group had outcomes superior to those of the exposure-alone group. Thus, cognitive interventions may have a special role in social phobia.

Heimberg et al. (1988) also studied a group of carefully diagnosed social phobics. Thirty-nine such individuals were divided into two groups:
one received cognitive-behavioral treatment (Heimberg et al., 1987), and
the other underwent educational/support group therapy. Both groups dis-
played improvement after treatment and at six-month follow-up. However, the cognitive-behavioral group showed significantly more improvement on most of the posttest measures and achieved a 75 percent overall
improvement rating, substantially higher than the 42 percent improvement rate of the educational support group. At six-month follow-up the
respective improvement rates were judged to be 80 and 50 percent. Like
the Butler et al. (1984) study, this report suggests a strong role for cognitive interventions in treating social phobia.

In general, cognitive-behavioral therapy has not been as widely used
for anxiety as for depression. This may be due to the fact that many studies of anxiety have tested individual cognitive interventions, as opposed
to testing whole cognitive-behavioral treatment packages (Stravynski and
Greenberg, 1987; Clark and Beck, 1988). What is evident from the literature is that cognitive-behavioral interventions seem to add little to the
treatment of simple phobia or OCD compared to exposure-based treatments. Cognitive-behavioral therapy does show promise in the treatment
of social phobia. However, its usefulness with PTSD has not been established due to the lack of controlled studies.

TREATMENT OF ANXIETY: A GENERAL MODEL

Treatment of anxiety disorders has become more sophisticated, especially
in agoraphobia and, more recently, in panic disorder (Barlow, 1988). Increased research on anxiety has contributed to the development of manuals allowing more consistent therapy (Mathews et al., 1981; Beck et al.,
1985; Barlow and Cerny, 1988). Also, the distinction between behavioral
and cognitive methods in treating anxiety is less important than the use
of a researched package of interventions combining both methods (Barlow 1988).

Treatment of Anxiety: Aversion Model

The remainder of this chapter focuses on a generic model for the treatment of anxiety. This model does not offer specific interventions for DSM
III-R anxiety disorders but serves as a starting point in developing a treatment plan for patients with such disorders. For specific interventions, the
reader is directed to more extensive works (Mathews et al., 1981; Beck
et al., 1985; Steketee and Foa, 1985; Barlow, 1988; Barlow and Cerny,
1988).

The literature on cognitive-behavioral therapy of depression suggests
that teaching a concrete, understandable rationale may be the significant

mediating factor in successful treatment (Kornblith et al., 1983). It is reasonable to extend that philosophy to the treatment of anxiety. A complete rationale should explain the physiological as well as the cognitive aspects of anxiety. Also, the rationale must predict how the individual will respond to different situations, especially in the exposure aspect of treatment.

The description of treatment as a coping model will set the stage for collaborative work between therapist and patient (Beck et al., 1985; Clark and Beck, 1988). This description must include discussions of (1) belief in the uncertainty or uncontrollability of anxiety; (2) vulnerability to danger symbols; (3) location of danger cues (internal vs. external); and (4) time dimensions (present vs. future danger [anticipatory anxiety]) (Beck et al., 1985; Barlow, 1988). Also emphasized are the role of cognitions, affect, physiological changes, and the way in which these three components facilitate the establishment of a vicious cycle of anxiety.

The literature shows that exposure to the feared situation is a key component in treatment (Barlow, 1988). However, there are two other components that are important clinically in treating anxiety: coping skills dealing with the physical aspect of anxiety (e.g., relaxation) and cognitive integration (e.g., cognitive restructuring). It must be noted that these last two components are helpful but not sufficient in treating anxiety disorders.

Controlling Physical Aspects of Anxiety

Relaxation has long been accepted as beneficial in a wide variety of problems (Barlow and Cerny, 1988), and in treating anxiety this can be an important part of a multicomponent treatment package. However, the choice of procedure (e.g., progressive muscle relaxation, guided imagery) depends on the individual being treated. Relaxation has been shown to be one of the better entry points in treating anxiety; it is easy to introduce and gives some immediate relief of symptoms.

For some individuals, though, relaxation will not be helpful in coping with physical aspects of anxiety; in these cases, distraction techniques may be useful alternatives. These techniques encourage the patient to shift from an internal focus on the increase in physical sensations to an external focus on concrete action. Examples include describing in detail the contents of a purse or briefcase, counting backward from 100 by seven, or doing multiplication tables (for more examples, see Beck et al., 1985).

Patients may also use controlled breathing to cope with the physical aspects of anxiety, particularly symptoms of panic or panic attacks (Salkovskis et al., 1986). This enables individuals to understand their role in the physical aspects of anxiety or panic. Overbreathing during a therapy session demonstrates how this alone increases a variety of physical symptoms (dry mouth, rapid heartbeat, dizziness, etc.). Controlled breathing is then shown to be a tool that decreases these physical symptoms. Usually individuals are taught to breathe at a rate of 8 to 12 breaths per minute. They are then told to practice at home (via an audiotape) and to use the controlled breathing as they experience changes in physical symptoms. This method has been shown to decrease panic and has become part of the treatment for panic attacks (Clark, 1986).

Cognitive interventions assist in changing and integrating the experience of anxiety (Borkovec et al., 1987). They also build an understanding of the role of anxiety in both normal and abnormal situations. Cognitive-behavior therapy usually starts with behavioral interventions and then moves progressively to cognitive procedures. However, behavioral interventions continue throughout treatment.

Most cognitive treatments for anxiety are taken from several different sources, including Antaki and Brewin (1982), Beck and Emery (1979), McKay et al. (1981), and Sank and Shaffer (1984). However, the work of Beck (Beck et al., 1979, 1985) gives a more comprehensive view of cognitive procedures. These generally consist of the following in some combination: (1) Socratic questioning; (2) monitoring and recording thoughts during anxious periods; (3) generating alternatives or adaptive responses to these thoughts; (4) training the patient to give a new meaning to the anxiety situation's reattribution training; and (5) identification of cognitive errors.

Exposure, either imaginal or in vivo, is fundamental to the treatment of anxiety (Barlow, 1988). Indirect exposure presents the fear-inducing cues to the imagination, usually in a hierarchical manner and often paired with relaxation. Direct measures involve prolonged exposure to the fear-inducing situation, usually with the personal assistance of the therapist. Ideally, the individual remains in the feared situation until anxiety diminishes. Direct exposure can also be presented in a graded or hierarchical fashion, and a self-paced approach is developed by the therapist and the individual during a session. This exposure is then applied outside the session with the patient and the therapist, and progress is discussed during the next session.

Studies on the length and intensity of exposure show variable results (Barlow, 1988). However, it seems that gradual exposure is more effective than intensive exposure. Also, the use of a fear hierarchy developed by the patient may be more effective over time. Most important is the individual's pursuit of exposure outside the office setting (Barlow, 1988).

SUMMARY

At present, exposure is still the most widely accepted treatment for anxiety. No current cognitive therapy for anxiety has been widely acccepted by clinicians (Beckham and Watkins, 1989). Hopefully, the current availability of treatment manuals will foster research clarifying the role of cognitive therapy in the treatment of anxiety. This will be especially important, since early research suggests that cognitive therapy may be very useful in the treatment of social phobia.

REFERENCES

American Psychiatric Association: *Diagnostic and Statistical Manual of Mental Disorders,* ed 3, rev. Washington, DC: American Psychiatric Association, 1987.
Antaki C, Brewin C (eds): *Attributional and Psychological Change.* London, Academic Press, 1982.
Barlow DH: *Anxiety and Its Disorders.* New York, Guilford Press, 1988.
Barlow DH, Beck JG: The psychosocial treatment of anxiety disorders: Current status, future directions, in Williams JBW, Spitzer RL (eds): *Psychotherapy Research: Where Are We and Where Should We Go?* New York, Guilford Press, 1984, pp 29–66.
Barlow DH, Cerny JA: *Psychological Treatment of Panic.* New York, Guilford Press, 1988.
Beckham EE, Watkins JT: Process and outcome in cognitive therapy, in Freemen A, Simon K, Beutler LE, et al (eds), *Comprehensive Handbook of Cognitive Therapy.* New York, Plenum Press, 1989, pp 61–82.
Beck AT: *Cognitive Therapy and the Emotional Disorders.* New York, International Universities Press, 1976.
Beck AT, Emery G: *Cognitive Therapy of Anxiety and Phobic Disorders.* Philadelphia, Center for Cognitive Therapy, 1979.
Beck AT, Emery G, Greenberg RL: *Anxiety Disorders and Phobias: A Cognitive Perspective.* New York, Basic Books, 1985.
Beck AT, Rush AJ, Shaw BF, et al: *Cognitive Therapy of Depression.* New York, Guilford Press, 1979.
Biran M, Augusto F, Wilson GT: In vivo exposure vs. cognitive restructuring in the treatment of scriptophobia. *Behav Res Ther* 19:525–532, 1981.
Biran M, Wilson GT: Treatment of phobic disorders using cognitive and exposure methods: A self-efficacy analysis. *J Consult Clin Psychol* 49:886–899, 1981.
Black JL, Keane TM: Implosive therapy in the treatment of combat related fears in World War II veterans. *J Behav Ther Exp Psychiatry* 13:163–165, 1982.
Borkovec TD, Mathews AM, Chambers A, et al: The effects of relaxation training with cognitive therapy or nondirective therapy and the role of relaxation-induced anxiety in the treatment of generalized anxiety. *J Consult Clin Psychol* 55:883–888, 1987.
Bourque P, Ladouceur R: An investigation of various performance-based treatments with acrophobics. *Behav Res Ther* 18:161–170, 1980.
Butler G, Cullington A, Munby M, et al: Exposure and anxiety management in the treatment of social phobia. *J Consult Clin Psychol* 52:642–650, 1984.
Clark DM: A cognitive approach to panic. *Behav Res Ther* 24:461–470, 1986.
Clark DM, Beck AT: Cognitive approaches, in Last CG, Hersen M (eds): *Handbook of Anxiety Disorders* New York, Pergamon Press, 1988, pp 362–385.

Deffenbacher JL, Suinn RM: Generalized anxiety disorder, in Michelson L, Ascher LM (eds): *Anxiety and Stress Disorders: Cognitive-Behavioral Assessment and Treatment*. New York, Guilford Press, 1987, pp 332–360.

Ellis A: *Reason and Emotion in Psychotherapy*. New York, Lyle Stuart, 1962.

Emmelkamp PMG: *Phobic and Obsessive-Compulsive Disorders: Theory, Research, and Practice*. New York, Plenum Press, 1982.

Emmelkamp PMG: Behavior therapy with adults, in Garfield SL, Bergin AC (eds): *Handbook of Psychotherapy and Behavior Change*. New York, John Wiley & Sons, 1986, pp 385–442.

Emmelkamp PMG, van der Helm M, van Zanten BL, et al: Contributions of self-instructional training to the effectiveness of exposure *in vivo:* A comparison with obsessive-compulsive patients. *Behav Res Ther* 18:61–66, 1980.

Emmelkamp PMG, Visser S, Hoekstra RJ: Cognitive therapy vs. exposure in vivo in the treatment of obsessive-compulsives. *Cogn Ther Res* 12:103–114, 1988.

Fairbank JA, Gross RT, Keane TM: Treatment of posttraumatic stress disorder: Evaluating outcome with a behavioral code. *Behav Modification* 7:557–568, 1983.

Foa EB, Grayson JB, Steketee G, et al: Success and failure in the behavioral treatment of obsessive-compulsive. *J Consult Clin Psychol* 15:287–297, 1983.

Foa EB, Steketee GS, Ozarow BJ: Behavior therapy with obsessive-compulsive: From theory to treatment, in Mavissakalian M, Turner SM, Michelson L (eds): *Obsessive-Compulsive Disorders: Psychological and Pharmacological Treatment*. New York, Plenum Press, 1985, pp 121–140.

Foy DW, Donahoe CP, Carroll EW, et al: Posttraumatic stress disorder, in Michelson L, Ascher LM (eds): *Anxiety and Stress Disorders: Cognitive-Behavioral Assessment and Treatment*. New York, Guilford Press, 1987, pp 361–378.

Hayes SL, Hussain RA, Turner AE, et al: The effect of coping statements on progress through a desensitization hierarchy. *J Behav Ther Exp Psychiatry* 14:117–129, 1983.

Heimberg RG, Dodge CS, Becker RE: Social phobia, in Michelson L, Ascher LM (eds): *Anxiety and Stress Disorders: Cognitive-Behavioral Assessment and Treatment*. New York, Guilford Press, 1987, pp 280–309.

Heimberg RG, Dodge CS, Hope DA, et al: Cognitive behavioral group treatment for social phobia: Comparison to a credible placebo control. Manuscript submitted for publication, in Barlow DH (ed): *Anxiety and Its Disorder: The Nature and Treatment of Anxiety and Panic*. New York, Guilford Press, 1988, pp 533–564.

Keane TM, Kaloupek DG: Imaginal flooding in the treatment of a post-traumatic stress disorder. *J Consult Clin Psychol* 50:138–140, 1982.

Kenny FT, Mowbray RM, Lalani S: Faradic disruption of obsessive ideation in the treatment of obsessive neurosis: A controlled study. *Behav Ther* 9:209–221, 1978.

Kipper DA: Behavior therapy for fears brought on by war experiences. *J Consult Clin Psychol* 45:216–221, 1977.

Kornblith SJ, Rehm LP, O'Hara MW, et al: The contribution of self-reinforcement training and behavioral assignments to the efficacy of self-control therapy for depression. *Cogn Ther Res* 7(6):499–528, 1983.

Kuch K, Swinson RP, Kirby M: Posttraumatic stress disorder after car accidents. *Can J Psychiatry* 30:426–427, 1984.

Ladouceur G: Participant modeling with or without cognitive treatment for phobias. *J Consult Clin Psychol* 51:942–944, 1983.

Last CG: Simple phobia, in Michelson L, Ascher LM (eds): *Anxiety and Stress Disorders: Cognitive-Behavioral Assessment and Treatment*. New York, Guilford Press, 1987, pp 176–190.

Liebowitz MR, Gorman JM, Feyer AJ, et al: Social phobia: Review of a neglected anxiety disorder. *Arch Gen Psychiatry* 42:729–736, 1985.

Linden W: Exposure treatments for focal phobias. *Arch Gen Psychiatry* 38:769–775, 1981.

Marshall WL, Segal Z: Behavior therapy, in Last CG, Hersen M (eds): *Handbook of Anxiety Disorders*. New York, Pergamon Press, 1988, pp 338–361.

Mathews A, Gelder MG, Johnston DW: *Agoraphobia: Nature and Treatment*. New York, Guilford Press, 1981.

Mavissakalian M, Barlow DH (eds): *Phobia: Psychological and Pharmacological Treatment*. New York, Guilford Press, 1981.

McKay M, Davis M, Fanning P: *Thoughts and Feelings: The Art of Cognitive Stress Intervention*. Richmond, Va., New Harbinger Press, 1981.

Meichenbaum D: *Cognitive-Behavior Modification*. New York, Plenum Press, 1977.

Meyer V: Modification of expectations in cases with obsessional rituals. *Behav Res Ther* 4:273–280, 1966.

Ost LG, Jerremalm A, Johannsson J: Individual response patterns and the effects of different behavior methods in the treatment of social phobia. *Behav Ther Res* 19:1–16, 1981.

Rachman SJ, Hodgson RS: *Obsessions and Compulsions*. Englewood Cliffs, NJ: Prentice-Hall, 1980.

Saigh PA: In vitro flooding of childhood post-traumatic stress disorders: A systematic replication. *Professional School Psychol* 2:133–144, 1987.

Salkovskis PM, Jones DRO, Clark DM: Respiratory control in the treatment of panic attacks: Replication and extension with concurrent measurement of behaviour and pCO_2. *Br J Psychiatry* 148:526–532, 1986.

Sank LJ, Shaffer CS: *A Therapist's Manual for Cognitive Behavior Therapy in Groups*. New York, Plenum Press, 1984.

Solomon Z, Benbenishty R: The role of proximity, immediacy, and expectancy in frontline treatment of combat stress reaction among Israelis in the Lebanon war. *Am J Psychiatry* 1436:613–617, 1986.

Solyum L, Kingstone E: An obsessive neurosis following morning glory seed ingestion treated by aversion relief. *J Behav Ther Exp Psychiatry* 4:293–295, 1973.

Steketee G, Foa EB: Obsessive-compulsive disorder, in Barlow DH (ed): *Clinical Handbook of Psychological Disorders*. New York, Guilford Press, 1985, pp 69–144.

Stravynski A, Greenberg D: Cognitive therapies with neurotic disorders: Clinical utility and related issues. *Compr Psychiatry* 28:141–150, 1987.

Trower P, Yardley K, Bryant D, et al: The treatment of social failure: A comparison of anxiety-reduction and skills acquisition procedures on two social problems. *Behav Modification* 2:41–60, 1978.

Vermilyea BB, Barlow DH, O'Brien GT: The importance of assessing treatment integrity: An example in the anxiety disorders. *J Behav Assessment* 6:1–11, 1984.

Williams SL, Dooseman G, Kleifield E: Comparative effectiveness of guided mas-
    tery and exposure treatments for intractable phobias. *J Consult Clin Psychol*
    52:505–518, 1984.
Williams SL, Turner SM, Peer DF: Guided mastery and performance desensiti-
    zation treatments for severe acrophobia. *J Consult Clin Psychol* 53:237–247,
    1985.

4

Treatment of Panic Disorder and Agoraphobia

JAMES C. BALLENGER

Effective treatment of panic disorder and agoraphobia has evolved in essentially two parallel lines since the early 1960s and includes both pharmacological and nonpharmacological treatments. The effective nonpharmacological treatments are primarily behavioral, although cognitive therapy has recently shown promise. Effective pharmacological treatments began with the tricyclic and monoamine oxidase inhibitor antidepressants and now include the benzodiazepine-type drugs. Pharmacological and nonpharmacological treatments are employed both singly and in combination. This chapter will first discuss the nonpharmacological treatments, their features, and estimates of their efficacy. It will then consider antidepressant and benzodiazepine-type treatments of panic disorder, focusing on how to use the medications, their side effects, estimates of their efficacy, and comparisons between medications. The chapter will close with a brief discussion of the relationship between nonpharmacological and pharmacological treatments.

NONPHARMACOLOGICAL TREATMENTS

Behavioral Therapies

Exposure in Imagination

Probably the first widely used behavioral treatment was systematic desensitization (SD), initially described by Wolpe (1969). In this technique, patients are first instructed in a relaxation technique, often deep muscle relaxation. They then construct a hierarchy of the situations they fear, and in therapy they pair images of these phobic situations with relaxation. During treatment the patients imagine their phobic scenes, working up from the least frightening to the most frightening. Before imagining the phobic stimulus, the patients are made to relax. They then imagine the phobic scene until they can imagine it without anxiety. Next, they move on to a more frightening scene.

This technique has generally proven relatively ineffective when compared to newer techniques (Gelder and Marks, 1966). Zitrin and colleagues (Zitrin et al., 1978) compared SD for 26 sessions, with and without imipramine, to supportive therapy and imipramine. They reported that SD in combination with imipramine was no more effective than supportive therapy and imipramine, although it was more effective than SD and placebo. However, Gelder and colleagues (1973) found SD to be as effective as flooding in imagination and flooding in vivo and significantly more effective than a control group.

Flooding in Imagination

In this technique, the patient and therapist construct scenes of phobic situations and then present them in imagination, but without pairing exposure with relaxation. The scenes are held in imagination until anxiety decreases. The patients are presented images of their phobic situations until none of the scenes produce anxiety. Marks and colleagues (1971) demonstrated that flooding in imagination was significantly better than SD, and these improvements were sustained at one year follow-up. Approximately two-thirds of the patients in these studies were agoraphobic. In a group of agoraphobics, Chambless and colleagues (1979) compared flooding in imagination, with and without methohexitone, for eight sessions compared to an attention control group. There was marked improvement in the flooding group but no change in the control group, and flooding under the influence of methohexitone was significantly less effective than flooding alone.

Emmelkamp and Wessels (1975) compared flooding in imagination to real-life exposure (see below) and found no differences between the two treatments. Also, flooding in fantasy coupled with real-life exposure was demonstrated to be effective in multiple studies (Gelder et al., 1973; Stern and Marks, 1973; Emmelkamp, 1974).

Direct Exposure

According to Marks (1973) and others (Leitenberg, 1976), reexposure in real life to the phobic situation is the principal curative factor in effective behavioral treatments. Apparently, methods that directly expose patients to phobic situations are the most efficient and probably the most effective (Marks, 1973). Exposure treatments vary from gradual exposure—a progression from the least frightening to the most frightening situations over a period of time—to total flooding—a direct, rapid confrontation with the phobic situation. Techniques also vary from therapist-assisted to family- or spouse-assisted to homework exposure, which is accomplished by the patient alone or with other phobics. In each type, patients are encouraged to enter the phobic situation and remain there until their anxiety level falls significantly. In graded exposure (Hafner and Marks, 1976; Mathews et al., 1976), patients may be asked to walk to the street outside the clinic, walk to a market and shop briefly, and take progressively longer rides on a public conveyance, all the while increasing the distance from their support person, place, or therapist. Marks states that these sessions should be longer than one hour for maximum improvement (Stern and Marks, 1973).

Mathews and colleagues (1976) compared real-life exposure to flooding in imagination and demonstrated no significant differences during treatment or at six-month follow-up, though real-life exposure had greater immediate clinical effects (Johnston et al., 1976). However, other studies have demonstrated that exposure in vivo results in greater improvement than flooding in imagination. Emmelkamp and colleagues (1978) also found that in vivo exposure was more effective than cognitive treatment (see below). Recently, Michelson and colleagues (1985) reported a twelve-week comparison of graded exposure to relaxation therapy (RT) and paradoxical intention (PI) therapy in a study involving a total of 31 patients. All treatments were highly effective, but 100 percent of the ten patients in the graded exposure cell met the criteria for high end-stage functioning at the end of treatment compared to 50 percent of the RT and PI patients. Interestingly, this study demonstrated a loss of panic attacks in approximately 50 percent of the patients in each treatment cell.

Nontherapist-Assisted Exposure

Exposure treatments can be accomplished with relatively little assistance from a therapist. Exposure programs in which patients confront their phobic situations on their own have also been shown to be effective (Mathews et al., 1977; Jannoun et al., 1980). In fact, Mavissakalian and colleagues have demonstrated that exposure after patients read an instruction manual was effective in one-third of their sample. Instructions given by a therapist, a self-help type book, or even a computer appear to be equally effective (Ghosh and Marks, 1987). Barlow et al. (1980) have described spouse-assisted (after instruction from a therapist) in vivo exposure. Two of the three patients were markedly improved, and the improvement was maintained over a six-year follow-up period. Because of its efficiency, this type of exposure assistance is now widely employed, as is utilization of other phobics or recovered phobics to assist patients with homework exposure assignments.

Outcome of Behavioral Treatments
in Panic Disorder and Agoraphobia

Unfortunately, many of the studies reported above have not utilized clear inclusion criteria or standard diagnostic techniques and have not reported the percentage of agoraphobics in the samples studied. Also, exposure outside of formal treatment sessions has often not been recorded. Only recently have study designs clearly portrayed the clinical meaningfulness of reported results. Nonetheless, it is important to attempt an estimation of clinical results with behavioral treatment because its clinical use is so widespread. A research consensus conference sponsored by the National Institutes of Mental Health on anxiety disorders (Barlow and Wolfe, 1981) concluded that exposure-based treatments resulted in "substantial, clinically significant improvement in 65–75 percent of patients who complete treatment but approximately 50% if dropouts were included in the analysis." In a review of 24 controlled studies involving 652 agoraphobic patients, Jansson and Öst (1982) stated that reported improvement reached their criterion of clinical significance in 55 percent of patients in the outcome studies utilizing direct or combined exposure treatments. Approximately two-thirds of the patients in the direct exposure studies maintained this improvement at six months. Several outcome studies have shown continuing and at times enhanced improvement five to ten years after treatment (Emmelkamp and Kuipers, 1979; Munby and Johnston, 1980), although some have not (Munby and Johnston, 1980).

Thus, although many forms of behavioral therapy are effective in the treatment of agoraphobia, the extent of that improvement remains controversial. Most studies do not report what percentage of patients improve to the point where they are well or almost well. When that criterion ("high end-stage functioning") is utilized, many authorities in the behavioral therapy field feel that only 30 to 50 percent become "nearly asymptomatic" (Barlow, personal communication; Mavissakalian, 1988). This rate may not be significantly higher than that obtained with the simplest forms of behavioral therapy or even the placebo response rate in recent large pharmacological trials (Ballenger et al., 1988).

Many studies show clearly that pharmacological treatments (especially imipramine) enhance the efficacy of exposure treatments such that approximately 65–75 percent of patients reach a "nearly asymptomatic" state (Zitrin et al., 1980, 1983; Telch et al., 1985). What remains to be clearly demonstrated is the relative percentages of patients with marked improvement due to behavioral exposure treatments alone, in combination with medications, or with medications alone. An effort to accomplish this is currently in progress (R. Swinson, personal communication).

Cognitive Therapy

Cognitive therapy generally involves attempts to restructure cognitions related to anxiety-provoking situations. Cognitive restructuring generally involves (1) identification of abnormal anxiety-producing thoughts, (2) demonstration of their anxiety-producing effects, and (3) challenge of their validity (Walen et al., 1980; Jansson and Öst, 1982). In so-called self-instructional training, emphasis is placed on repeated practice to allow the phobic patient to think differently in phobic situations (Meichenbaum, 1977).

Emmelkamp and colleagues (1978), as described above, compared cognitive therapy to exposure in vivo for 12 agoraphobics and demonstrated that patients receiving cognitive therapy improved less than those treated with exposure. Recently, Barlow (1988) and Barlow and Craske (1988) described a treatment for panic disorder (without agoraphobia) that combines elements of cognitive therapy with desensitization to internal physical cues. Patients' beliefs that panic attacks involve dangerous physical changes are challenged first by systematic identification and then by a demonstration of their link to anxiety. Physiological symptoms similar to those experienced during anxiety episodes are simulated by various techniques (hyperventilation, spinning in a chair, etc.), and the patients are allowed to habituate to these symptoms through practice and cognitive restructuring. Preliminary results are very promising, with significant clinical improvement in over 80 percent of the patients treated and marked reduction of panic attacks. Although this study involved only a small number of patients the improvement seen with cognitive therapy alone was at least comparable to that of alprazolam alone.

PHARMACOLOGICAL TREATMENTS

Imipramine

Approximately a dozen double-blind, placebo-controlled studies have compared imipramine to placebo, with the majority demonstrating that imipramine is significantly superior in the treatment of panic disorder (see Lydiard and Ballenger, 1988, for a review). Although some controversy remains (Marks et al., 1983), most experts believe imipramine's effectiveness in panic disorder to be one of the best-established facts in psychopharmacology and consider it the "gold standard" against which new pharmacological treatments of panic disorder are measured (De la Fuente and Sepulveda, 1988; Klerman, 1988).

Oral Dosage

As many as one-third of patients experience an initial hyperstimulatory reaction, lasting for two to three weeks, especially to imipramine and desipramine. It is unpleasant and frightening to patients and, not uncommonly, leads to discontinuation of treatment. Many clinicians begin treatment with very low doses (e.g., 10 mg/day of imipramine) to reduce the occurrence of this side effect. Doses can then be increased every one to three days as tolerated. If this reaction does occur, it can usually be managed by reassurance, support, dose reduction, beta blockers, or benzodiazepines. Also, patients seem more tolerant of this side effect if they have been warned that it might occur beforehand and assured that it is harmless if it does occur.

Clinical experience has suggested that doses of 150 mg/day or more of imipramine are required for an optimal response in many patients. Recently, Mavissakalian and Perel (1985) provided evidence from a controlled trial that imipramine in doses lower than 150 mg/day is associated with response rates similar to those of placebo. However, if patients receive 150 mg/day or more (mean, 188 mg/day), they attain excellent clinical response rates; 65–95 percent of patients have responded quite well on various outcome measures.

Studies are also beginning to describe relationships between plasma levels of imipramine and desipramine and a clinical response. Ballenger and colleagues (1984) maintained one group of 18 panic disorder and agoraphobia patients at a serum level of 100–150 ng/ml of imipramine plus desmethylimipramine for three months and a second group of 18 patients at 200–250 ng/ml. Patients were also treated in weekly group therapy with exposure homework. Both groups responded significantly and had essentially identical responses, suggesting that the 100–150 ng/ml range was sufficient for most patients. In 15 agoraphobic patients, Mavissakalian and colleagues (1984) demonstrated a correlation of imipramine (but not desmethylimipramine or the combination) and a clinical response. Subsequent studies (Marks et al., 1983; Nesse et al., 1984; Aronson, 1987) have failed to observe a relationship between plasma levels and clinical response. However, the study of Marks et al. (1983) failed to observe an overall positive response to imipramine, and this would cloud any possible plasma level/clinical response relationship. Recently, Mavissakalian and colleagues, in a carefully designed, stratified dose study with imipramine, confirmed earlier work (Ballenger et al., 1984) suggesting that plasma imipramine levels of 100–150 ng/ml are required for an overall positive clinical response (Mavissakalian, 1988).

Length of Treatment

There are few systematic data concerning the optimal length of pharmacological treatment with imipramine, or any other medication for that matter. While most studies demonstrate that it takes three to six months for the acute response to be completed, there are no studies suggesting how much longer treatment should continue. Routine practice in many centers is to continue imipramine (or other medications) for a total of six to twelve months before considering attempts to discontinue this therapy. The general rationale for continued treatment is that patients need these additional months to consolidate the clinical gains in social and occupational areas before risking a relapse with medication discontinuation.

Monoamine Oxidase Inhibitor (MAOI) Antidepressants

In the early 1960s, evidence from open trials demonstrated that MAOI antidepressants were effective. The largest study, of approximately 250 patients, was that of Kelley et al. (1970), which demonstrated that the

MAOIs were effective in the large majority of patients. In a carefully per-formed trial in the late 1970s, patients received placebo, imipramine, or phenelzine (average dose, 55 mg/day) and biweekly group therapy ses-sions promoting exposure over a twelve-week period (Sheehan, et al., 1980); phenelzine was shown to be quite effective against the entire range of panic disorders. There are now at least six placebo-controlled trials of the MAOIs in panic disorder (Lydiard and Ballenger, 1987, 1988). Most have studied phenelzine, and although the evidence is somewhat less con-sistent and extensive than that for the tricyclic antidepressants, it is clear that the MAOI antidepressants are an effective treatment for panic dis-order.

Recently, Buigues and Vallejo (1987) reported strongly positive results with phenelzine in an open study of panic disorder patients with and with-out agoraphobia. They noted almost complete resolution of panic attacks and reduction of other symptoms with a mean dose of 55 mg/day over a treatment period of three to six months. In a recent open trial previously mentioned, Howell and colleagues (1987) observed strongly positive ef-fects in 18 patients receiving phenelzine (mean dose, 53.5 mg/day) and weekly group therapy promoting exposure over a twelve-week period. Sheehan (1986) has reported an unpublished trial comparing phenelzine to imipramine, alprazolam, and placebo, again with significant effects of phenelzine against panic attacks, phobic behavior, and disability second-ary to the phobic syndrome.

To our knowledge, the only controlled trial with tranylcypromine in recent years occurred in Brazil (Versiani et al., 1987). It found tranylcy-promine in a dose of 30 mg/day effective in over 90 percent of patients.

Clinical Use of MAOI

Treatment with phenelzine is generally initiated at a dose of 15 mg/day, increasing as tolerated to 45–60 mg/day. Some patients respond to lower doses and occasional patients appear to require 75–90 mg/day. During maintenance treatment, improvement is generally sustained if doses are reduced (e.g., to 30 mg/day) and side effects are decreased on these lower doses. All the MAOIs tend to cause insomnia; therefore, treatment is usu-ally initiated with divided doses given with breakfast and lunch. Side ef-fects generally resemble those seen with tricyclic antidepressants, and postural hypotension may be a particular problem.

Other Antidepressants

Controlled trials with other antidepressants are relatively limited. Lydiard (1987a) reported that panic disorder patients responded to desipramine at a dose of 200 mg/day for three to four months. He also reported that a plasma level above 150 ng/ml was associated with a greater likelihood of a positive response.

Recent studies suggest that several of the serotonin reuptake blocker antidepressants are effective in this disorder. There are at least three published, placebo-controlled trials demonstrating the efficacy of chlorimipramine (Escobar and Landbloom, 1976; Amin et al., 1977; Karabanow, 1977). A large but as yet unpublished comparative trial in Brazil likewise reported that chlorimipramine was effective (Versiani, 1987). Finally, Den Boer and colleagues (1987) found both chlorimipramine and fluvoxamine effective in the treatment of panic disorder. Zimelidine was more effective than placebo in a small trial by Evans and colleagues (1986), and fluoxetine seemed effective in an open trial by Gorman and colleagues (1987). Although Gorman et al. treated their patients with 20–40 mg/day, subsequent clinical experience has suggested that some patients should begin with less than 20 mg/day. The published studies on trazodone used in panic disorder have been mixed. In a study comparing trazodone to imipramine and alprazolam, Charney and colleagues (1986) found that trazodone was markedly less effective than the other two agents. However, in a small trial, Mavissakalian and colleagues (1987) reported much more favorable clinical effects.

Two reports (Muskin and Fyer, 1981; Lydiard, 1987b) indicate that maprotiline is effective, but one indicates that it is not (Den Boer and Westenberg, 1988). According to additional, anecdotal experience, nortriptyline, amitriptyline, and doxepin are also effective (Lydiard and Ballenger, 1987). Bupropion is the only agent that clearly seems ineffective (Sheehan et al., 1983), although, as mentioned, trazodone was demonstrated in one study to be less effective.

Relapse

The rate of patient relapse after antidepressants are discontinued is currently difficult to estimate accurately, but rates in most studies have ranged between 20 and 35 percent (Kelly et al., 1970; Zitrin and Klein, 1980, 1983; Zitrin et al., 1987). In stark contrast is the 70–90 percent relapse rate reported by Sheehan (1986) after treatment with imipramine, phenelzine, and alprazolam. However, Sheehan's definition of relapse required only the occurrence of two panic attacks, and this may have contributed to these high percentages. Although generally not specified in the other studies, the definition of relapse generally involved the reappearance of more symptoms than in the Sheehan trial. Relapse rates will be studied much more rigorously in current, ongoing trials, and more accurate estimates of relapse rates should be available in the next few years. It is fortunate that most clinicians find that patients who relapse after discontinuing medication have a very high response rate when medication is reinstituted, making attempts to gradually discontinue medication a rational and safe procedure. As discussed below, concomitant behavioral treatment may influence the risk for relapse in medication trials. Mavissakalian and Michelson (1986), for example, observed only minor losses in clinical efficacy over a two-year follow-up period in patients initially treated with three months of imipramine and exposure therapy.

Benzodiazepines

Traditional Benzodiazepines

Until recently, benzodiazepines were thought to be ineffective in the treatment of panic disorder with and without agoraphobia. This widespread conclusion probably resulted from the fact that most panic patients had taken benzodiazepines previously and reported that their symptoms had not substantially decreased. However, evidence from multiple clinical studies now indicates that many, if not most, of the benzodiazepines are effective. The most likely explanation for this confusion is that recent research trials have utilized daily use and adequate doses of the benzodiazepines.

The first indication that a benzodiazepine was effective in panic disorder was provided by a trial by McNair and Kahn (1981) in which chlordiazepoxide was compared to imipramine in 36 agoraphobic patients. Two papers then reported that the triazolobenzodiazepine alprazolam was effective in this condition. Chouinard and colleagues (1982) described a double-blind, placebo-controlled, eight-week trial in which alprazolam was effective in low doses of 0.5 to 3 mg/day (mean, 2.05 mg/day). Sheehan and colleagues (1984) quickly followed this with a single-blind trial comparing alprazolam and ibuprofen. Alprazolam patients given 2 to 6 mg/day (mean, 5.4 mg/day) improved significantly on patient and physician global ratings, and panic attacks and phobic anxiety were reduced. Alexander and Alexander (1986) reported that alprazolam in low doses (mean, 2.2 mg/day) led to remission of panic attacks in 85 percent of 27 patients seen in their clinical practice. Resolution of phobic avoidance behaviors also occurred in 93 percent of patients, but this generally required higher daily doses. The optimal dose for resolution of the full range of symptoms was around 4 mg/day, varying from 4.0–9.9 mg/day in 41 percent of the patients.

Based on these promising preliminary findings, the Upjohn Company sponsored a large multinational trial comparing alprazolam and placebo in panic disorder and panic disorder with agoraphobia. The trial occurred in two phases; the first compared alprazolam and placebo, and the second compared alprazolam to imipramine and placebo in a larger sample.

Phase I of this trial involved more than 500 patients, was the largest study ever conducted in the panic disorder field, and was the first large trial in this field to employ a medication-alone design, without any type of psychotherapy or behavior therapy. It was a double-blind, placebo-controlled, flexible-dose study performed in five centers in the United States, two in Canada, and one in Australia. Patients met DSM III criteria for either panic disorder (15 percent) or agoraphobia with panic attacks (85 percent), and all patients had had at least one panic attack during each of the previous three weeks. A total of 471 patients completed twenty-one days of treatment, with 92 percent of the alprazolam patients finishing the eight-week trial compared to 56 percent of those on placebo. Dropouts in the placebo group occurred primarily for ineffectiveness. The mean dose of alprazolam by week 8 was 5.7 ± 2.2 mg/day.

Alprazolam was significantly more effective than placebo on almost all outcome measures for each week, and its significant effects were apparent in the first week of treatment. At the primary comparison point in this trial (week 4), there were significant alprazolam/placebo differences in spontaneous and situational panic attacks, phobic fears, phobic avoidant behavior, anxiety, and secondary disability in work, social, and family life. Significantly more patients on alprazolam were markedly improved (35 percent vs. 10 percent) and moderately improved (52 percent vs. 33 percent) on the global outcome measures. By week 8, 51 percent of the alprazolam patients were markedly improved and 41 percent were moderately improved, compared to 37 percent and 26 percent of the patients remaining in the placebo cell. At week 4, 50 percent of the alprazolam patients and 28 percent of the placebo patients had eliminated their panic attacks, and the percentage of alprazolam patients that were panic free at week 8 had risen to 59 percent. At the beginning of the trial, 84 percent of the patients in both groups described their reaction to their main phobia as either "markedly or extremely fearful." By week 4, the percentage of alprazolam patients who had this level of fear had fallen to 38 percent, while 59 percent of the placebo patients remained that fearful. There were similar significant reductions in anxiety and disability in family and social life secondary to panic and phobic symptoms.

The response to alprazolam was surprisingly rapid, and almost one-half of the eventual improvement occurred in the first week. Improvement continued throughout the eight weeks of the trial, but this trial provided the first definitive evidence that the onset of action for alprazolam was more rapid than for the antidepressants.

Acceptance of alprazolam was high, and less than 5 percent of the patients dropped out because of side effects. The most common side effects were sedation, fatigue, slurred speech, ataxia, and amnesia. However, the side effects were generally managed easily by a transient reduction in dose or by slowing the increase in alprazolam.

Phase II of this trial compared alprazolam, imipramine, and placebo for eight weeks with a very similar patient group and study design. This trial took place in 12 different centers in Western Europe, the United States, and South America, with a total of 1,166 patients. The results of this trial have not yet been published but have been presented preliminarily (De la Fuente and Sepulveda, 1988).

Again, the attempt was made to treat patients with 6 mg/day of alprazolam and to compare the results obtained with 150 mg/day of imipramine. Alprazolam was effective during the first week and across all outcome measures. The effects of imipramine were not significant until approximately week 3 or 4 on most outcome measures, but by week 8, imipramine's clinical effects were generally not significantly different from those of alprazolam. The primary difference observed was the different speed in onset of action, but alprazolam was also better tolerated and resulted in significantly fewer dropouts.

Noyes et al. (1984) compared diazepam to propranolol. Seventeen patients on diazepam had a reduction of panic attacks from 8.5 to 2.9 per week during the second week, and 86 percent of those on diazepam (mean dose, 30 mg/day) showed moderate or marked improvement during the first two weeks of treatment, while only 33 percent improved to that degree on propranolol. Dunner and colleagues (1986) reported that diazepam (mean, 44 mg/day) reduced panic attacks from a mean of 3.3 to 0.6 per week ($n = 13$) over six weeks; In this trial, the effects of diazepam and alprazolam were roughly comparable.

As mentioned, McNair and Kahn (1981) gave 36 panic disorder patients chlordiazepoxide (mean, 55 mg/day) or imipramine (mean, 132 mg/day) for an eight-week trial and found imipramine significantly superior. However, chlordiazepoxide was also shown to be effective in this trial, a result replicated in the 1986 study of Khan et al.

Second-Generation Benzodiazepines

Demonstration that alprazolam was effective led to several subsequent studies to determine whether other second-generation benzodiazepines were also effective. Howell and colleagues (1987) reported their preliminary results comparing lorazepam to phenelzine in panic disorder patients in a flexible-dose open trial. Twenty-two patients were treated with each medication for a period of three months, and all patients received concomitant behavioral therapy in a group therapy setting. Both medications were approximately equal in efficacy. Clinical improvement in panic attacks and other phobic symptoms was apparent in the first one to two weeks with lorazepam but only after four to six weeks with phenelzine. In this trial, the mean dose of lorazepam was 3.8 ± 1.3 mg/day.

Charney and colleagues (1987) have presented data on 48 panic disorder patients in which lorazepam was compared to alprazolam in a double-blind six-week trial. Treatment with both medications resulted in significant and roughly equivalent improvement, which was evident in the first week. A multicenter, double-blind study comparing lorazepam and alprazolam was recently presented (Charney et al., 1987). This was an eight-week trial of 102 patients; again, both treatment groups had significant and similar improvement across the full range of panic and phobic symptoms. After six weeks, 83 percent of the alprazolam-treated patients and 90 percent of the lorazepam-treated patients reported moderate to marked improvement on global ratings. Side effects occurred in 60–70 percent of patients in both groups, and there were no significant differences in clinical efficacy or side effects.

Beaudry et al. (1984) reported that bromazepam was effective in a single case.

In a series of uncontrolled studies, it was suggested that clonazepam, a high-potency benzodiazepine often used in the treatment of certain types of epilepsy, was also effective in panic disorder. Chouinard and colleagues (Chouinard et al., 1983; Fontaine and Chouinard, 1984) reported that clonazepam was effective in 10 of 12 patients with panic disorder or agoraphobia with panic attacks. Recently, the Massachusetts General Hospital group in Boston (Spier et al., 1986) reported their retrospective analysis of the first 50 patients they treated with clonazepam. In this group, 22 patients had panic disorder and 28 had panic disorder with agoraphobia. The average dose of clonazepam was 1.9 ± 1.0 mg/day (range, 0.75 to 6.0 mg/day). Of the 44 patients who completed two weeks of treatment, 78 percent responded, with the average drop in global ratings (CGI) falling from the markedly ill to the moderately ill range to the borderline mentally ill to the normal range. Interestingly, 41 patients had previously failed to respond to other medications, and three-fourths of them responded to clonazepam.

There are two ongoing control trials comparing clonazepam to alprazolam by Chouinard in Canada and by Rosenbaum and colleagues at the Massachusetts General Hospital. An interim analysis of the Rosenbaum et al. comparison of clonazepam and alprazolam demonstrated significant drug-placebo differences but little differences between the two medications (Pollack et al., 1987). In this trial, the mean dose was 2.4 mg/day for clonazepam and 5.2 mg/day for alprazolam.

Other Agents

Although promising in generalized anxiety disorder, buspirone was shown in one trial to be no more effective than placebo and significantly less effective than imipramine (Sheehan et al., 1987). However, buspirone was shown to be effective in isolated case reports, and its use might be reasonable when other agents have failed.

Propranolol, a commonly used beta blocker, has been employed to treat panic disorder patients and does reduce some of the distressing cardiovascular side effects associated with panic disorder. It has also been useful in patients with antidepressants that produce anticholinergic side effects and increases in heart rate. However, to this point, placebo-controlled clinical trials have not provided convincing evidence that beta blockers are as useful as other agents in the overall treatment of panic disorder (Noyes, 1985; Noyes et al., 1984).

Carbamazepine appears to have limited therapeutic efficacy in acute patients (Klein et al., 1987). However, other anecdotal evidence suggests that it may have wider usefulness, and confirmation will have to await controlled trials. Similarly, verapamil (Klein and Uhde, 1988) and valproic acid (Primeau and Fontaine, 1988) may have limited antipanic effects in small numbers of patients.

Comparative Trials of Pharmacological Treatments

The only published comparative trial between a tricyclic and a MAOI was the imipramine-phenelzine-placebo comparison by Ballenger et al. (1977) and Sheehan et al. (1980). Phenelzine was more effective than imipramine on almost every outcome measure, and on the two most important behavioral outcome measures, phenelzine was significantly more effective than imipramine. In his unpublished comparison of imipramine-phenelzine-alprazolam-placebo, Sheehan (1986) noted trends favoring phenelzine over imipramine, though none of the differences reached statistical significance. Moreover, Ballenger and colleagues (1987) compared phenelzine to alprazolam, imipramine, and lorazepam, all combined with self-exposure homework and weekly group therapy. They too noted significantly greater efficacy for phenelzine on several measures. In other comparisons, as mentioned, Charney and colleagues (1986) reported that imipramine was superior to trazodone, and Evans and colleagues (1986) found that zimelidine was superior to both imipramine and placebo. Also, as mentioned, Versiani et al. (1987) recently found few differences between chlorimipramine, imipramine, tranylcypromine and alprazolam.

Comparisons Between Antidepressants and Benzodiazepine-Type Agents

Perhaps the earliest report comparing an antidepressant to a benzodiazepine demonstrated that imipramine was more effective than chlordiazepoxide in blocking panic attacks (McNair and Kahn, 1981). Most of the remaining trials have compared imipramine to alprazolam. Two double-blind, placebo-controlled trials (Matuzas et al., 1986; Rizley et al., 1986) found both medications to be effective and essentially equivalent, although alprazolam's effects became significant in the first week of treatment, while those of imipramine required four to eight weeks. In one trial, alprazolam patients experienced significantly greater global improvement, reduction in panic and nonpanic anxiety, and fewer side effects (Rizley et al., 1986). Alprazolam patients reported feeling more alert and vigorous, while imipramine patients reported a reduction in anger. These results are quite similar to those of the open trials by Charney et al. (1986) and Ballenger and colleagues (1987) in finding relatively few differences between medications except speed of onset. Similarly, the double-blind comparison of imipramine, phenelzine, and alprazolam by Sheehan (1986), as previously mentioned, found few differences between alprazolam and both antidepressants, as did the large trial by Versiani et al. (1987). The most definitive comparison between alprazolam and imipramine is the recently completed Phase II of the Cross National Panic Study, which compared alprazolam, imipramine, and placebo. As previously discussed, in that trial of almost 1,200 patients, alprazolam was again found to have significant effects in the first week of treatment and was significantly superior to imipramine for the first four weeks of treatment (De la Fuente and Sepulveda, 1988). However, by week 8, imipramine and alprazolam both had significant effects and were no different from each other. These initial differences and ultimate similarities in clinical effects were seen across all symptom measures and represent some of the most definitive results in this field.

There are only a few trials that allow comparison between benzodiazepines. In the two trials that compared alprazolam and lorazepam (Ballenger et al., 1987; Charney et al., 1987), and alprazolam and clonazepam (Tesar et al., 1987), there were few differences between the medications in terms of clinical efficacy or side effects.

Clinical Use of the Benzodiazepines

The most common side effects reported with the use of benzodiazepines are sedation and ataxia, which occur in approximately one-third of the patients in most trials. Usually, these side effects are easily managed by slowing dosage increases or reducing the dose transiently. Side effects rarely necessitate discontinuation of the benzodiazepines. In fact, one of the principal differences between antidepressant and benzodiazepine treatment of panic disorder has been the significantly larger group of patients who remain on benzodiazepines compared to tricyclics. In general, patients tolerate all of the benzodiazepines well.

Rare serious side effects of the benzodiazepines include episodes of depression with alprazolam (Lydiard et al., 1987), lorazepam (Howell et al., 1987), and clonazepam (Spier et al., 1986). It is not clear that these depressions were secondary to benzodiazepine use, but in several reports, depressive symptoms were reduced after the benzodiazepine dose was lowered. Several incidents of irritability and verbal aggression were reported with the benzodiazepines, and hepatic abnormalities were reported in 2 patients in the Phase I alprazolam trial (247 alprazolam patients), but there were no reports of hepatic difficulties in the subsequent larger trial (386 alprazolam patients).

Use of benzodiazepines is generally well accepted by patients and clinicians. Patients are not as apprehensive about taking benzodiazepines as they are about taking tricyclics. In the initial weeks of antidepressant treatment, approximately one-third of the patients have the so-called hyperstimulation reaction, with increases in anxiety, tachycardia, palpitations, and a "speeded-up" sensation. Patients' increased initial acceptance of benzodiazepines compared to antidepressants is generally related to an awareness of this possibility, often from previous experience with very short courses of antidepressants. Physicians appear to have accepted the use of benzodiazepines widely because of their rapid onset of action, ease of administration, and favorable side effects spectrum, especially when compared to the antidepressants.

DISCONTINUATION PHENOMENA

Symptoms of physiological dependence and return of symptoms secondary to relapse occur in some patients when medications are discontinued. In fact, withdrawal symptoms can be severe (e.g., seizure) if benzodiazepines are discontinued suddenly (Brier et al., 1984; Noyes, 1985). It is difficult to estimate accurately the incidence and severity of withdrawal symptoms in panic disorder patients because most of the data available are from uncontrolled studies, generally with alprazolam. This area of research is also complicated by frequent and rapid relapse as benzodiazepines are tapered, in contrast to the slower relapse (and initial recovery) when antidepressants are utilized. Symptoms of relapse and withdrawal are quite similar and at times indistinguishable.

Although the data are limited, a group of patients (126) from the Phase I alprazolam-placebo trial was studied in a placebo-controlled withdrawal phase that followed treatment (Pecknold et al., 1988). One-third (35 percent) of patients experienced a transient withdrawal syndrome, as well as transient rebound increases in panic attacks and other symptoms. The majority of patients showed increases in symptoms in the last week of discontinuation of alprazolam and in the first week after it was stopped. However, by the end of the second week following taper, the level of symptoms fell to that observed in the placebo group. The issues of withdrawal, relapse, and rebound are important in the overall risk/benefit analysis of the benzodiazepines and are currently under investigation in several well-designed studies.

It is probably important to point out that many patients and their families, and even their physicians, have considerable fear of the physiological or psychological dependence resulting from the use of benzodiazepines. Patients often express a fear of becoming addicted to or dependent on the medications. On questioning, their fear is often that they will not be able to manage their symptoms without the medication, and this reduced sense of control and lowered self-esteem at times result in patients discontinuing effective medications. Panic disorder patients have very similar concerns about both antidepressants and benzodiazepines, but benzodiazepine use often raises special questions and concerns for their physicians and society. These issues are often confused with issues of drug abuse. However, reports of the abuse of benzodiazepines in panic disorder patients are rare (Juergens and Moise, 1988) and almost invariably involve patients who are abusing illegal drugs and utilizing the benzodiazepines to reduce the adverse effects of those drugs.

PHARMACOTHERAPY COMBINED WITH BEHAVIORAL THERAPY

Unfortunately, there is still no definitive trial in which an effective behavioral therapy is compared to an effective pharmacotherapy and both compared to the combination of the two. Only this design would allow a comprehensive analysis of the relative efficacy of these three alternatives.

However, there are studies that have attempted systematically to examine the contribution of pharmacological treatment to behavioral treatments. Most of them have suggested that behavioral treatments and pharmacotherapy (generally with imipramine) are more effective than behavioral treatments alone or medication alone (Mavissakalian et al., 1983). In fact, Telch and colleagues (1985) replicated their finding that instructions to avoid exposure to phobic situations significantly interfered with the efficacy of imipramine. When compared to agoraphobics on imipramine alone (mean, 125 mg/day), those on imipramine plus self-exposure homework for 12 weeks experienced significantly greater improvement. Similarly, Mavissakalian and Michelson (1986) found that behavioral treatment combined with imipramine was significantly superior to behavioral treatment alone. Klein and his co-workers (1987) reanalyzed data from their two large imipramine studies (Zitrin et al., 1980, 1983) and reported that exposure does reduce phobic avoidance behavior but not panic frequency, and that imipramine reduces the frequency of both panic attacks and phobic avoidance. A large comparison of behavioral therapy alone, medication alone, and a combination of the two is currently underway. While we await the results, most clinical experience and the data cited above suggest that the most effective treatment for panic disorder and agoraphobia is probably a combination of medication and behavioral exposure treatments. However, this remains a topic of considerable controversy primarily involving those behavior therapists who feel that panic disorder is best treated by nonpharmacological behavioral methods. While it has not been studied, many believe that the most commonly offered treatments presently are behavioral therapy alone, medication alone, or, most frequently, a combination of pharmacotherapy and exposure therapy.

It has frequently been argued that behavioral treatments for panic disorder are superior to pharmacological treatments because clinical improvements are maintained or even enhanced after behavioral treatments but are lost after pharmacological treatments. While it certainly appears true that the improvements seen with behavioral exposure treatments used alone are generally maintained (Marks, 1973; Michelson et al., 1985) and that significant loss of improvement can occur when medication alone is utilized (Sheehan, 1986), this does not appear to be the case if medications are combined with exposure treatments. Cohen and colleagues (1984) have reported that two-year follow-up after treatment with behavioral therapy plus either imipramine or placebo demonstrated that approximately two-thirds of the patients treated with behavioral therapy and placebo or imipramine continued to maintain substantial improvement. Similarly, approximately two-thirds of the patients described by Mavis-sakalian and Michelson (1986) were doing well after two years. These patients had initially received imipramine or placebo, flooding exposure therapy, programmed exposure, or a combination and, although there was some loss of efficacy in the imipramine cells and some enhancement in the exposure cells, group mean changes were small, did not reach significance, and certainly did not reflect a return to pretreatment levels. This trial (Mavissakalian and Michelson, 1986) is perhaps the clearest one in the literature demonstrating what might be expected in terms of relative clinical response from modern exposure behavioral treatments alone and exposure combined with imipramine. Thus, in the twelve-week acute treatment phase of this trial, the percentage of patients with a marked clinical response ("high end-stage functioning") was as follows: imipramine plus flooding = 64 percent, imipramine plus programmed exposure = 65 percent, flooding alone = 47 percent, and programmed exposure alone = 29 percent. As mentioned, over the next six months there were no significant differences between the treatment groups. In two-thirds of all patient groups, agoraphobia was "no longer a problem." The improvements were also similarly maintained in all groups at the two-year follow-up. The authors speculate that the concomitant exposure treatment may have contributed to the high maintenance of imipramine improvement. It is also likely that the acute differences favoring imipramine would have been maintained had its use been continued.

There is considerable consensus across trials combining medications and some form of exposure therapy that 65 to 75 percent of patients have a marked response to this regimen. This suggests that an excellent clinical response can be obtained and maintained in at least two-thirds of the patients treated with combined imipramine and exposure therapy if the initial response is maximized by the use of 150 mg/day or more of imipramine and if adequate doses of imipramine are continued. However, the optimal length of treatment and the relapse rate are yet to be determined.

REFERENCES

Alexander PE, Alexander DD: Alprazolam treatment for panic disorders. *J Clin Psychiatry* 47:301–304, 1986.

Amin MM, Ban TA, Pecknold JC, et al: Chlorimipramine (Anafranil) and behavior therapy in obsessive-compulsive and phobic disorders. *J Int Med Res* 5(5):33–37, 1977.

Aronson TA: A naturalistic study of imipramine in panic disorder and agoraphobia. *Am J Psychiatry* 144:1014–1019, 1977.

Ballenger JC, Burrows G, DuPont RL Jr, et al: Alprazolam in panic disorder and agoraphobia: Results from a multicenter trial. I. Efficacy in short-term treatment. *Arch Gen Psychiatry* 45(5):413–422, 1988.

Ballenger JC, Howell EF, Laraia MT, et al: Comparison of four medications in panic disorder. Presented at the annual meeting of the American Psychiatric Association, Chicago, May 9–14, 1987.

Ballenger JC, Peterson GA, Laraia M, et al: A study of plasma catecholamines in agoraphobia and the relationship of serum tricyclic levels to treatment response, in Ballenger, JC (ed): *Biology of Agoraphobia*. Washington, DC, American Psychiatric Association Press, 1984, pp 27–64.

Ballenger JC, Sheehan DV, Jacobson GC: Antidepressant treatment of severe phobic anxiety. Presented at the annual meeting of the American Psychiatric Association, Toronto, May 2–6, 1977.

Barlow DH: *Anxiety and Its Disorders: The Nature and Treatment of Anxiety and Panic*. New York, Guilford Press, 1988.

Barlow DH, Craske M: Cognitive treatment of panic disorder. Presented at the International Behavior Therapy Conference, Edinburgh, Scotland, November 1988.

Barlow DH, Mavissakalian MR, Schofield LD: Patterns of desynchrony in agoraphobia: A preliminary report. *Behav Res Ther* 18:441–448, 1980.

Barlow DH, Wolfe BE: Behavioral approaches to anxiety disorders: A report on the NIMH-SUNY Albany Research Conference. *J Consult Clin Psychol* 49:448–454, 1981.

Beaudry P, Fontaine R, Chouinard G: Bromazepam, another high potency benzodiazepine for panic attacks. *Am J Psychiatry* 141:464–465, 1984.

Brier A, Charney DS, Nelson CJ: Seizures induced by abrupt discontinuation of alprazolam. *Am J Psychiatry* 141:1606–1607, 1984.

Buigues J, Vallejo J: Therapeutic response to phenelzine in patients with panic disorder and agoraphobia with panic attacks. *J Clin Psychiatry* 48:55–59, 1987.

Chambless DL, Foa EB, Groves GA, et al: Flooding with brevital in the treatment of agoraphobia: Countereffective? *Behav Res Ther* 17:243–251, 1979.

Charney DS, Woods SW, Goodman WK, et al.: The efficacy of lorazepam in panic disorder. Presented at the 140th Annual Meeting of the American Psychiatric Association, Chicago, NR 165, 110, 1987.

Charney DS, Woods SW, Goodman WK, et al: Drug treatment of panic disorder: The comparative efficacy of imipramine, alprazolam, and trazodone. *J Clin Psychiatry* 47:580–586, 1986.

Chouinard G, Annable L, Fontaine R, et al: Alprazolam in the treatment of generalized anxiety and panic disorders: A double-blind, placebo-controlled study. *Psychopharmacology* 77:229–233, 1982.

Chouinard G, Labonte A, Fontaine R, et al: New concepts in benzodiazepine therapy: Rebound anxiety and new indications for more potent benzodiazepines. *Prog Neuropsychopharmacol Biol Psychiatry* 7:669–673, 1983.

Cohen S, Montiero W, Marks IM: Two-year follow-up of agoraphobia after exposure and imipramine. *Br J Psychiatry* 144:276–281, 1984.

De la Fuente JR, Sepulveda J: Drug treatment of panic anxiety. Presented during the symposium "Treatment of Anxiety Disorders" at the 141st annual meeting of the American Psychiatric Association, Montreal, May 8, 1988.

Den Boer JA, Westenberg HG: Effect of a serotonin and noradrenaline uptake inhibiting panic disorder: A double-blind comparative study with fluvoxamine and maprotiline. *Int Clin Psychopharmacol* 3(1):59–74, 1988.

Den Boer JA, Westenberg HGM, Kamerbee WD, et al: Effect of serotonin uptake inhibitors in anxiety disorders: A double-blind comparison of clomipramine and fluvoxamine. *Int Clin Psychopharmacol* 2:21–32, 1987.

Dunner DL, Ishiki D, Avery DH, et al: Effect of alprazolam and diazepam on anxiety and panic attacks in panic disorder: A controlled study. *J Clin Psychiatry* 47:458–460, 1986.

Emmelkamp PMG: Self-observation versus flooding in the treatment of agoraphobia. *Behav Res Ther* 12:229–237, 1974.

Emmelkamp PMG, Kuipers AC: Agoraphobia: A follow-up study four years after treatment. *Br J Psychiatry* 134:352–355, 1979.

Emmelkamp PMG, Kuipers ACM, Eggeraat JB: Cognitive modification versus prolonged exposure in vivo: A comparison with agoraphobics as subjects: *Behav Res Ther* 16:33–41, 1978.

Emmelkamp PMG, Wessels H: Flooding in imagination vs. flooding in vivo: A comparison with agoraphobics. *Behav Res Ther* 13:7–15, 1975.

Escobar JI, Landbloom RP: Treatment of phobic neurosis with chlorimipramine: A controlled clinical trial. *Cur Ther Res* 20:680–685, 1976.

Evans L, Kenardy J, Schneider P, et al: Effect of a selective serotonin uptake inhibitor in agoraphobia with panic attacks: A double-blind comparison of zimelidine, imipramine, and placebo. *Acta Psychiatr Scand* 73:49–53, 1986.

Fontaine R, Chouinard G: Antipanic effects of clonazepam. *Am J Psychiatry* (letter to editor) 141:149, 1984.

Gelder MG, Bancroft JHJ, Gath DH, et al: Specific and non-specific factors in behavior therapy. *Br J Psychiatry* 123:445–462, 1973.

Gelder MG, Marks IM: Severe agoraphobia: A controlled prospective trial of behaviour therapy. *Br J Psychiatry* 112:309–319, 1966.

Ghosh S, Marks IM: Self-directed exposure for agoraphobia: A controlled trial. *Behav Ther* 18(1):3–16, 1987.

Gorman JM, Liebowitz MR, Fyer AJ, et al: An open trial of fluoxetine in the treatment of panic attacks. *J Clin Psychopharmacol* 7:329–332, 1987.

Hafner J, Marks I: Exposure in vivo of agoraphobics: Contribution of diazepam, group exposure, and anxiety evocation. *Psychol Med* 6:71–88, 1976.

Howell EF, Laraia MT, Ballenger JC, et al: Lorazepam treatment of panic disorder. Presented at the annual meeting of the American Psychiatric Association, Chicago, May 9–14, 1987.

Jannoun L, Munby M, Catalan J, et al: A home-based treatment program for agoraphobia: Replication and controlled evaluation. *Behav Ther* 11:294–305, 1980.

Jansson L, Öst LG: Behavioral treatments for agoraphobia: An evaluative review. *Clin Psychol Rev* 2:311–336, 1982.

Johnston DW, Lancashire M, Mathews AM, et al: Imaginal flooding and exposure to real phobic situations: Changes during treatment. *Br J Psychiatry* 129:372–377, 1976.

Juergens SM, Moise RM: Alprazolam dependence in seven patients. *Am J Psychiatry* 145(5):625–627, 1988.

Kahn RJ, McNair DM, Lipman RS, et al: Imipramine and chlordiazepoxide in depressive and anxiety disorders. II. Efficacy in anxious outpatients. *Arch Gen Psychiatry* 43:79–85, 1986.

Karabanow O: Double-blind controlled study in phobias and obsessions. *Int J Med Res* 5:42–48, 1977.

Kelly D, Guirguis W, Frommer E, et al: Treatment of phobic states with antidepressants: A retrospective study of 246 patients. *Br J Psychiatry* 116:387–398, 1970.

Klein DF, Ross DC, Cohen P: Panic and avoidance in agoraphobia: Application of path analysis to treatment studies. *Arch Gen Psychiatry* 44:377–385, 1987.

Klein E, Uhde TW: Controlled study of verapamil for treatment of panic disorder. *Am J Psychiatry* 145:431–434, 1988.

Klein E, Uhde TW, Post RM: Carbamazepine, alprazolam withdrawal, and panic disorder: Reply to letter. *Am J Psychiatry* (letter to editor) 144:266, 1987.

Klerman GL: Overview of the cross-national collaborative panic study. *Arch Gen Psychiatry* 45:407–412, 1988.

Leitenberg H: Behavioral approaches to treatment of neuroses, in Leitenberg, H (ed): *Handbook of Behavior Modification and Behavior Therapy*. Englewood Cliffs, NJ, Prentice-Hall, 1976, pp 124–167.

Lydiard RB: Desipramine in agoraphobia with panic attacks: An open, fixed-dose study. *J Clin Psychopharmacol* 7:258–260, 1987a.

Lydiard RB: Successful utilization of maprotiline in a patient intolerant of tricyclics. *J Clin Psychopharmacol* 7:113–114, 1987b.

Lydiard RB, Ballenger JC: Antidepressants in panic disorder and agoraphobia. *J Affect Dis* 13:153–168, 1987.

Lydiard RB, Ballenger JC: Panic-related disorders: Evidence for efficacy of the antidepressants. *J Clin Psychiatry* 49(1):17–19, 1988.

Lydiard RB, Laraia MT, Ballenger JC, et al: Emergence of depressive symptoms in patients receiving alprazolam for panic disorder. *Am J Psychiatry* 144:664–665, 1987.

Marks IM: Reduction of fear: Towards a unifying theory. *Can Psychiatr Assoc J* 18:9–12, 1973.

Marks IM, Boulougouris J, Marset P: Flooding versus desensitization in the treatment of phobic patients. A crossover study. *Br J Psychiatry* 119:353–375, 1971.

Marks IM, Gray S, Cohen D, et al: Imipramine and brief therapist-aided exposure in agoraphobics having self-exposure homework. *Arch Gen Psychiatry* 40:153–162, 1983.

Mathews AM, Johnston DW, Lancashire M, et al: Imaginal flooding and exposure to real phobic situations: Treatment outcome with agoraphobic patients. *Br J Psychiatry* 129:362–371, 1976.

Mathews A, Teasdale J, Munby M, et al: A home-based treatment program for agoraphobia. *Behav Ther* 8:915–924, 1977.

Matuzas W, Uhlenhuth EH, Glass RM, et al: Alprazolam and imipramine in panic disorder: a life table analysis. Presented at the annual meeting of the American College of Neuropsychopharmacology. Washington, D.C., Dec. 8–12, 1986.

Mavissakalian M: Clinical response relationship to serum levels of imipramine. Presented at the annual meeting of the Phobia Society of America, Boston, November 1988.

Mavissakalian M, Michelson LL: Agoraphobia: relative and combined effectiveness of therapist-assisted in vivo exposure and imipramine. *J Clin Psychiatry* 47:117–122, 1986.

Mavissakalian M, Michelson L, Dealy RS: Pharmacological treatment of agoraphobia: Imipramine versus imipramine with programmed practice. *Br J Psychiatry* 143:348–355, 1983.

Mavissakalian M, Perel JP: Imipramine in the treatment of agoraphobia: Dose–response relationships. *Am J Psychiatry* 142:1032–1036, 1985.

Mavissakalian M, Perel J, Bowler K, et al: Trazodone in the treatment of panic disorder and agoraphobia with panic attacks. *Am J Psychiatry* 144:785–787, 1987.

Mavissakalian M, Perel J, Michelson L: The relationship of plasma imipramine and *N*-desmethyl-imipramine to improvement in agoraphobics. *J Clin Psychopharmacol* 4:36–40, 1984.

McNair DM, Kahn RJ: Imipramine compared with a benzodiazepine for agoraphobia, in Klein DF, Rabin J, ed: *Anxiety: New Research and Changing Concepts.* New York, Raven Press, 1981, pp 69–80.

Meichenbaum D: *Cognitive Behavior Modification: An Integrative Approach.* New York, Plenum Press, 1977.

Michelson L, Mavissakalian M, Marchione K: Cognitive and behavioral treatments of agoraphobia: Clinical, behavioral, and psychophysiological outcomes. *J Consult Clin Psychol* 53(6):913–925, 1985.

Munby M, Johnston DW: Agoraphobia: The long-term follow-up of behavioural treatment. *Br J Psychiatry* 137:418–427, 1980.

Muskin PR, Fyer AJ: Treatment of panic disorder. *J Clin Psychopharmacol* 1:81–90, 1981.

Nesse RM, Cameron OG, Curtis GC, et al: Adrenergic function in patients with panic anxiety. *Arch Gen Psychiatry* 41:771–776, 1984.

Noyes R, Jr: Beta-adrenergic blocking drugs in anxiety and stress. *Psychiatr Clin North Am* 8:119–132.

Noyes R Jr, Anderson DJ, Clancy J, et al: Diazepam and propanolol in panic disorder and agoraphobia. *Arch Gen Psychiatry* 41:287–292, 1984.

Pecknold JC, Swinson RP, Kuch K, et al: Alprazolam in panic disorder and agoraphobia: Results from a multicenter trial. III. Discontinuation effects. *Arch Gen Psychiatry* 45:429–436. 1988.

Pollack M, Rosenbaum JF, Tesar G, et al: Alprazolam versus clonazepam in panic disorders, in New Research Program and Abstracts, 140th Annual Meeting of the American Psychiatric Association, Chicago, NR167, 111, 1987.

Primeau F, Fontaine R: GABAergic agents and panic disorder. *Biol Psychiatry* 24:941–960, 1988.

Rizley R, Kahn RJ, McNair DM, et al: A comparison of alprazolam and imipramine in the treatment of agoraphobia and panic disorder. *Psychopharmacol Bull* 22:167–172, 1986.

Sheehan DV: Tricyclic antidepressants in the treatment of anxiety disorders. Presented at the annual meeting of the American Psychiatric Association, Washington, D.C., May 10–16, 1986.

Sheehan DV, Ballenger JC, Jacobsen G: Treatment of endogenous anxiety with phobic, hysterical, and hypochondriacal symptoms. *Arch Gen Psychiatry* 37:51–59, 1980.

Sheehan DV, Coleman JH, Greenblatt DJ, et al: Some biochemical correlates of panic attacks with agoraphobia and their response to a new treatment. *J Clin Psychopharmacol* 4:66–75, 1984.

Sheehan DV, Davidson J, Manschreck T, et al: Lack of efficacy of a new antidepressant (bupropion) in the treatment of panic disorder with phobias. *J Clin Psychopharmacol* 3:28–31, 1983.

Sheehan DV, Raj A, Soto S, et al: Is buspirone effective in the treatment of panic disorder? Presented at the annual meeting of the National Collaborative Drug Evaluation Unit, Key Biscayne, Florida, May 25–28, 1987.

Spier SA, Tesar GE, Rosenbaum JF, et al: Treatment of panic disorder and agoraphobia with clonazepam. *J Clin Psychiatry* 47:238–242, 1986.

Stern R, Marks I: Brief and prolonged flooding. A comparison in agoraphobic patients. *Arch Gen Psychiatry* 28:270–276, 1973.

Telch M, Agras WS, Taylor CB, et al: Combined pharmacological and behavioral treatment for agoraphobia. *Behav Res Ther* 23:325–335, 1985.

Tesar GE, Rosenbaum JF, Pollack MH, et al: Clonazepam versus alprazolam in the treatment of panic disorder: Interim analysis of data from a prospective double-blind, placebo-controlled trial. *J Clin Psychiatry* 48(10):16–19, 1987.

Versiani M, Costa e Silva J, Klerman G: Treatment of panic disorder with clomipramine, alprazolam, imipramine, and tranylcypromine. Presented at the annual meeting of the American College of Neuropsychopharmacology, San Juan, Puerto Rico, December 1987.

Walen SR, DiGuseppe R, Wessler RL: *A Practitioner's Guide to Rational Emotive Therapy.* New York, Oxford University Press, 1980.

Wolpe J: *The Practice of Behavior Therapy.* New York, Pergamon Press, 1969.

Zitrin CM, Juliano M, Kahan M: Five-year relapse rate after phobia treatment. Presented at the annual meeting of the American Psychiatric Association, Chicago, May 9–14, 1987.

Zitrin CM, Klein DF, Woerner MG: Behavior therapy, supportive psychotherapy, imipramine, and phobias. *Arch Gen Psychiatry* 35:307–316, 1978.

Zitrin CM, Klein DF, Woerner MG, et al: Treatment of phobias. I. Comparison of imipramine hydrochloride and placebo. *Arch Gen Psychiatry* 40:125–138, 1983.

Zitrin CM, Klein DF, Woerner MG: Treatment of agoraphobia with group exposure in vivo and imipramine. *Arch Gen Psychiatry* 37:63–72, 1980.

5

Psychopharmacological Management of Social and Simple Phobias

MICHAEL R. LIEBOWITZ

This chapter focuses on the clinical management of social and simple phobias. Since psychosocial approaches to anxiety disorders are covered elsewhere in this volume, this chapter deals principally with psychopharmacological treatment techniques.

SOCIAL PHOBIA

Definition

DSM III-R defines social phobia as "a persistent fear of one or more situations in which the person is exposed to possible scrutiny by others and fears that he or she may do something or act in a way that will be humiliating or embarrassing." Examples given include fear of public speaking, eating or drinking in front of others, urinating in a public bathroom, speaking up in a public meeting, and conversing at a social gathering.

To qualify as a social phobia, the condition must be sufficiently severe that feared situations are either avoided or endured with dread. In addition, the phobic fears have to interfere with occupational functioning or with usual social activities or relationships, or there has to be marked distress about having the fear.

The affected individual must also recognize that his or her fear is excessive and unreasonable. If an Axis III (medical disorder) or another Axis I psychiatric disorder is present, the social phobic fear has to be unrelated to it, i.e., the fear is not of publicly having a panic attack as part of panic disorder, stuttering in someone with stuttering, or trembling in a person with Parkinson's disease.

DSM III-R also provides for the subcategorization of the generalized type of social phobia if the phobic fears include most social situations. DSM III suggested that most socially phobic patients had only one feared situation, and offered as examples such discrete performance fears as speaking, writing, eating, drinking, or urinating in public. In DSM III, more widespread social fears were consigned to the category of "avoidant personality disorder." This was a departure from Marks and Gelder's (1966) original concept of social phobia, which included patients with both specific social fears (speaking, signing a check, or eating in public) and those with more generalized forms of social anxiety (fears of initiating a conversation or dating). In DSM III-R patients with the generalized type of social phobia may also meet the criteria for avoidant personality disorder, in recognition of the fact that the boundary between these two entities is currently uncertain.

In a social or performance situation, social phobics experience tachycardia, sweating, trembling, leg weakness, and a desire to flee. They fear appearing foolish or incompetent and worry that others can perceive their nervousness, which adds to their feelings of anxiety and embarrassment. Distraction by physical and emotional symptoms impairs performance, which further adds to anxiety. Anxiety and fear, in turn, exacerbate physical symptoms, creating a positive feedback loop that continues to escalate. In the extreme case, the individual becomes so anxious that further performance becomes impossible, or he or she simply bolts from the social situation.

Differential Diagnosis

Social phobia has been ignored in many clinical settings because it has not been recognized as a distinct syndrome that is highly amenable to one or more specific forms of treatment. Three common ways that the diagnosis of social phobia is often missed are (1) to consider it as simply extreme shyness, a normal variant on a continuum of personality functioning; (2) to view it as a manifestation of avoidant personality disorder; or (3) to classify it as part of agoraphobia.

DSM III and III-R take a categorical approach to psychiatric diagnosis, with the implication that designated diagnostic categories represent pathophysiologically distinct entities. This does not totally negate a dimensional approach but rather supersedes it. That is, social phobic patients may in fact be at one end of a continuum of social anxiety, the other end of which is complete fearlessness in social or performance settings. Nevertheless, because of the symptoms and disability suffered by social phobics and the extreme psychophysiological processes they experience, designation of these individuals as suffering a distinct disorder has two advantages. First, it calls attention to a problem that has heretofore been ignored. As illustrated below, this has spurred both epidemiological and clinical studies. Second, treatment efforts are more readily directed at the problem once it has been identified as a distinct clinical entity; this too, as discussed further on, has been very fruitful.

Lumping social phobia, or even its generalized subtype, with avoidant personality disorder creates a different set of problems. The most exciting clinical developments in social phobia involve the recent demonstration of the treatment efficacy of pharmacotherapy (Liebowitz et al., 1988b) and cognitive behavior therapy (Heimberg et al., 1985). To the degree that personality disorder implies intrapsychic conflict and pathological defensive operations, insight-oriented psychotherapy rather than pharmacotherapy or behavior therapy is usually considered. Thus viewing social phobics as having a personality disorder rather than an anxiety disorder reduces the likelihood of their receiving useful treatment.

In addition, data exist to suggest overlap of social phobia and avoidant personality. Turner et al. (1986) compared patients with each diagnosis and found marked similarities in cognitive content and physiological reactivity. The two groups differed in that the avoidant personality patients had greater interpersonal sensitivity and poorer social skills. These findings are compatible with a formulation that regards many instances of avoidant personality disorder as simply a more severe form of social phobia. While these extreme social phobics may not respond as well to behavior therapy as social phobics who don't also meet the criteria for avoidant personality, they do seem to respond as well to pharmacotherapy, especially with monoamine oxidase inhibitors (MAOIs) (Deltito and Perugi, 1986; Liebowitz et al., 1986, 1988).

Social phobic patients become diagnostically intermingled with agoraphobics in two ways. In one situation, clinicians simply fail to consider or specifically query for the distinctive features of social phobia. A patient may report that he or she has anxiety attacks and is reluctant to leave home, and is then diagnosed as agoraphobic with panic attacks when in fact the problem is social phobia. There are several important symptomatic distinctions. The agoraphobic with panic attacks begins having anxiety attacks unexpectedly. These attacks never become confined to a specific stimulus, although, as the illness progresses, certain situations can be identified in which they are more likely to occur. In addition, the agoraphobic would much rather go out accompanied than alone, and prefers to venture into a place where other people will be present to help if a disabling anxiety attack occurs. In contrast, social phobics develop anxiety attacks only when interacting with or being viewed by other people, or in anticipation of such an event. If they are fearful of going out, it is because they will meet or be seen by others and feel uncomfortable. In contrast to the agoraphobic, a social phobic would rather venture out alone than accompanied, would rather go out at night than during the day (less visibility), and would rather ride on an empty train or bus than on one with other people. Thus the individual with anxiety attacks and travel fears must be closely questioned on these issues to make the proper differential diagnosis.

In the second situation, investigators until recently, saw no reason to separate agoraphobics from social phobics in psychopharmacological investigations (see Liebowitz et al., 1985, for a review of this literature). Consequently, while studies demonstrated the efficacy of a drug like phenelzine in a combined agoraphobic-social phobic sample, it was impossible to know if the drug actually helped social phobia. Only recently have psychopharmacological trials focused on social phobics per se. This is important because we have reason to believe that there are differences in pharmacological responsivity between agoraphobics and social phobics. While both groups seem to respond to MAOIs (Sheehan et al., 1980; Liebowitz et al., 1988b), agoraphobics with panic attacks do well on tricyclics (Zitrin et al., 1983), while anecdotally, social phobics do not. However, controlled trials or tricyclics in social phobia are needed.

Magnitude of the Problem

The extent of the problems engendered by social phobia involve consideration of prevalence, age of onset and chronicity, and morbidity.

In a 1971 questionnaire survey, Bryant and Trower estimated that 3–10 percent of first-year students at a British college manifested typical social phobia. Looking at the general population, the Epidemiological Catchment Area (ECA) study found a six-month prevalence of social phobia in two U.S. urban areas of 0.9 to 1.7 percent for men and 1.5 to 2.6 percent for women (Myers et al., 1984). Most recently, using phone screening for four specific forms of social phobia in St. Louis, Pollard and Henderson (1988) found that 22.6 percent of the adult population had marked fear and/or avoidance of public speaking/performing, writing in front of others, eating in restaurants, or using public restrooms. However, less than 1 in 10 of these, or 2 percent of the population surveyed, also experienced marked distress or had distinct social or occupational impairment from these fears, thus fulfilling all of the social phobia criteria.

These data suggest several things. First, a sizable proportion of the general population, perhaps 2 percent, suffers some form of social phobia. Second, a much larger segment of the population has many of the problems of social phobia but learns to live with or adapt to them, so that affected individuals do not feel unduly distressed or impaired. Third, men may tolerate social phobic features less well than women, because while women comprise the majority in epidemiological samples (Myers et al., 1984), men comprise the majority in clinical samples (Liebowitz et al., 1985, 1988b). This is probably due to the fact that social phobia interferes more with male than female social and vocational roles as defined in our society, creating a greater incentive for males to overcome the problem.

In terms of morbidity, social phobia seems to begin early (characteristically before age 25 and usually before age 20) and to follow a chronic, unremitting course (Marks and Gelder, 1966; Aimes et al., 1983; Thyer et al., 1985). Vocational and social impairment are often significant. In one series, 2 of 11 patients were unable to work, 2 dropped out of school, 6 were blocked from work advancement, and 5 avoided almost all social interaction outside their immediate family (Liebowitz et al., 1985).

Significant depressive symptoms are also quite common in social phobics; among the 11 patients cited above, 5 had either past or present secondary major depression. In one large series one-half of the patients had significant depressive symptoms and 14 percent had a history of "parasuicidal acts" (Aimes et al., 1983). Social phobics frequently become depressed because of the obstacles experienced in trying to advance vocationally or expand socially.

Social phobic symptoms are also frequently found among alcoholics, usually predating the drinking problem (Mullaney and Trippett, 1979; Smail et al., 1984). Looking at the problem in reverse, one study found that 20 percent of social phobics consumed excessive amounts of alcohol, considerably more than the 7 percent of agoraphobics who did so (Aimes et al., 1983). Anecdotally, some social phobic patients reported that they felt the need to consume alcohol prior to their first evaluation in our anxiety disorders treatment program. The concurrence of social phobia and alcoholism complicates treatment efforts, because socially phobic alcoholics find the socialization of Alcoholics Anonymous aversive, while alcoholic social phobics often experience hepatic toxicity with MAOIs.

Pharmacotherapy of Social Phobia

As with any psychiatric disorder, adequate pharmacotherapy must be administered in the context of a solid therapeutic relationship. The treating pharmacotherapist must be, and appear to be, knowledgeable about social phobia in particular and anxiety disorders in general, as well as conversant with the benefits and potential adverse effects of the many available medications. Whether the pharmacotherapist is the sole treating professional or working adjunctively with a psychotherapist, time should be taken to establish rapport, review the patient's difficulties, and develop realistic medication treatment goals and timetables.

This said, classes of medication with some demonstrated efficacy to date include MAO inhibitors, beta blockers, and benzodiazepines.

MAO Inhibitors

The evidence for MAOI efficacy in social phobia consists of (1) pre-1985 treatment studies of mixed agoraphobic-socially phobic populations; (2) MAOI studies of the related entity of atypical depression; (3) open clinical reports with phenelzine and tranylcypromine; and (4) placebo-controlled phenelzine trials of discrete socially phobic populations.

As reviewed in detail elsewhere (Liebowitz et al., 1985), prior to 1985, four studies had found MAOIs superior to tricyclics in mixed agoraphobic-socially phobic populations. Because results were not reported separately for the social phobic subsample, clinicians could not be sure that the MAOIs were useful for this patient group. This ambiguity did provide an incentive, however, to investigate the matter further.

Another precursor to controlled MAOI studies in social phobia were MAOI-tricyclic comparisons in atypical depression (Liebowitz et al., 1984). Atyical depressives were defined as patients who met the requirements for a depressive syndrome and, in addition, exhibited mood reactivity (the ability to be temporarily cheered by pleasant events) and some constellation of overeating, oversleeping, extreme fatigue, and chronic interpersonal hypersensitivity. It is this last feature in particular that links atypical depressives to social phobics. Interpersonal hypersensitivity is the tendency to experience one's intereactions with others in an especially negative fashion by magnifying and/or being especially hurt by major as well as minor rejections, rebuffs, inattentions, or disappointments. We think of atypical depressives as very rejection sensitive; when experiencing severe interpersonal disappointment, especially of a romantic kind, the atypical depressive is plunged into a depressed, socially withdrawn state. The social withdrawal is usually episodic, and the patient resumes a more normal social life when the mood state lifts. However, after repeated romantic disappointments, for example, an atypical depressive may become chronically socially or at least romantically avoidant. In addition, some of these patients exhibit an avoidance of heterosexual intimacy that extends back to adolescence, in that sense closely resembling socially phobic patients.

Both social phobics, particularly the generalized subtype, and atypical depressives, are highly sensitive to emotional injury by others. In the atypical depressive, this leads to recurrent or chronic depressive states and episodic social withdrawal; in the social phobic, it leads to chronic social withdrawal and often episodic depression. Phenelzine treatment resulted in substantial improvement in approximately 70 percent of an atypical depressive sample in a six-week controlled comparison, as opposed to 50 percent for imipramine treatment and 30 percent for placebo. Moreover, the MAOI was far more effective than the other treatments in reducing interpersonal hypersensitivity, again suggesting its efficacy in social phobia.

As a next step, we conducted an open clinical trial of phenelzine in social phobia (Liebowitz et al., 1986). Eleven patients who met the DSM III criteria for social phobia were treated with phenelzine, starting at 30 mg/day and increasing by 15 mg/day/week to a maximum of 90 mg/day. Seven showed marked improvement within four to six weeks. As an example, a 19-year-old male at baseline avoided all performance and social encounters; as a consequence, he was unable to work or attend school. In fact, he generally avoided going out of the house except at night, when chance social encounters were less frequent, and he found interacting with the supermarket cashier so painful that he was unable to shop for things he wanted to buy.

The patient underwent several years of psychotherapy, which had no significant impact on his social fears. A prior trial with a beta blocker (described below) had been partially helpful, allowing him to return to school and take a part-time job, but he still remained fearful of participating in class or interacting with peers. When the beta blocker was stopped, he began to relapse and again contemplated quitting school and his job. Phenelzine was then started according to protocol. After four weeks on the MAOI, the patient appeared calmer and more appropriately assertive in social situations. He was able to attend school comfortably and continue his part-time job. In addition, for the first time, he was able to ask questions in class and ask girls for dates. This patient, as well as others, generally tolerated the phenelzine well, with the usual range of minor MAOI side effects.

Patients seemed sensitive to the dose of the MAOI, feeling overstimulated on too high a dose and insufficiently helped when the dose was too low. The effective dose varied among patients, however, ranging from 30 to 75 mg/day in this pilot trial and up to 90 mg/day in other patients.

Two other open clinical reports are important to note. Deltito and Perugi (1986) reported a patient with social phobia and avoidant personality disorder whose avoidant features (except for mild residual public speaking anxiety) virtually disappeared with phenelzine treatment. This result reinforces the point made before that severe generalized social phobia may merge indistinguishably with avoidant personality disorder and that the whole constellation may respond to MAOIs.

In addition, Versiani et al. (1988) have recently reported an open trial of tranylcypromine in 32 patients who met the DSM III criteria for social phobia. Excluding three early dropouts, 18 (62 percent) members of the sample were rated as markedly improved and 5 (17 percent) were rated as moderately improved at the end of two to three months of treatment. In this study, marked improvement was defined as the ability to face all performance and/or social situations with slight or no discomfort. A moderate response involved improved functional ability but continuing anxiety symptoms. These data suggest that MAOI efficacy in social phobia includes tranylcypromine as well as phenelzine. Interestingly, Versiani's group is now comparing phenelzine and placebo with the investigational reversible MAOI A inhibitor moclobomide in social phobia; the results are not yet available.

These promising results with MAOIs prompted a placebo-controlled trial of phenelzine in social phobia. Since the beta blocker atenolol was also included in that investigation, we will first review the earlier data for beta blockers in social phobia and then discuss the MAOI-beta blocker comparative study.

Beta Blockers

Numerous analogue studies have examined the effect of beta blockers on anxiety during observed performance in nonpatient samples. Of 11 trials reviewed (Liebowitz et al., 1985), 8 found a beta blocker superior to placebo in reducing some aspect of performance anxiety. Since the majority of these studies involved administration of short-term doses prior to a performance situation, the findings are most relevant to those social phobics who experience only occasional and predictable anxiety episodes, such as those accompanying public speaking or auditioning. In fact, the use of beta blockers to relieve undue anxiety accompanying public speaking or performing is widespread, suggesting at least some beneficial effects.

To pursue this topic further, we initiated an open clinical trial of the cardioselective, mainly peripherally acting beta blocker atenolol in 10 patients who met the DSM III criteria for social phobia (Gorman et al., 1985). The sample was mixed with regard to subtype, containing patients with discrete public speaking difficulties as well as those with more generalized social fears. All patients reported palpitations and sweating as prominent symptoms. Overall, five patients experienced marked improvement (relief of almost all social phobic symptoms and avoidance), and four others reported moderate improvement (reduced avoidance with some continued excessive fear) on atenolol, 50–100 mg/day taken daily over a six-week period. Contrary to expectations, marked improvement was not confined to patients with public speaking anxiety.

This result led us to include an atenolol treatment group in our placebo-controlled trial of phenelzine and placebo in social phobia. However, we already knew of one negative beta blocker study in which propranolol and placebo were compared in 16 social phobics, all of whom were concomitantly receiving social skills training (Falloon et al., 1981). The dose of propranolol was adjusted to lower the heart rate to 60/minute. No significant differences were noted between the six patients who received the beta blocker and the six who received placebo. Limitations of this study, however, included small sample size, lack of specific diagnostic criteria, blind ratings for social skills training, and the fact that four patients had panic attacks.

Controlled Phenelzine-Atenolol Comparison
in Social Phobia

This study has just been completed but has not yet been fully analyzed. The sample includes 87 patients with the DSM III criteria for social phobia who participated in at least the first eight-week phase of a phenelzine-atenolol-placebo comparison. Responders continued to be tested under double-blind conditions for another eight-week maintenance phase to assess the durability of the response. Continued responders to one of the active drugs were then gradually tapered and evaluated blind to the drug they were taking to assess whether continued treatment was needed to maintain clinical gains.

Data are currently available for 59 patients who entered the trial. Six of these responded to placebo during a prerandomization single-blind placebo washout, and six others dropped out during this phase (Liebowitz et al., 1988b). Of the remaining 47 patients randomized to one of the three treatments, 41 completed the eight-week acute treatment phase or were treated long enough (at least twenty-one days) to qualify for endpoint analyses. Six others dropped out during the first three weeks of randomized treatment (three on phenelzine, two on atenolol, and one on placebo).

Included among the 41 acute-phase completers were 14 on phenelzine, 11 on atenolol, and 16 on placebo. Defining a responder as someone with a week 8 or endpoint Clinical Global Impression (CGI) change score of much or very much improved, response rates were 64 percent (9/14) for phenelzine, 36 percent (4/11) for atenolol, and 31 percent (5/16) for placebo. While these proportions did not differ significantly, phenelzine was significantly superior to placebo on week 8 global severity and change ratings and significantly better than atenolol on the global change rating. These comparisons utilized analyses of covariance for severity scores (with baseline ratings as covariates) and analyses of variance for change scores.

The week 8 or end-of-phase mean atenolol dose was 95 mg, with a range of 50–100 mg. The mean phenelzine dose at the end of the acute phase was 72 mg/day, with a range of 45–90 mg/day. There were no significant differences in dose for either drug between responders and nonresponders.

Results from the first half of this placebo-controlled study suggest the efficacy of phenelzine but not atenolol in social phobia. These results are being maintained in the second half of the study as well, so that in the study as a whole, phenelzine but not atenolol has been found superior to placebo. Interestingly, however, when we look at the drugs' effect within the social phobic subtype (a designation of which was made prospectively), a more complicated picture emerges. Phenelzine appears more effective in the generalized subtype than in the discrete subtype of social phobia. Since most of the patients had the generalized form, this would account for phenelzine's superiority in the sample as a whole. Atenolol, on the other hand, is no better than placebo for the generalized subtype but appears helpful for the discrete form of social phobia.

This finding makes sense in light of what we know about the pathophysiology of social phobia. Two recent studies suggest that discrete social phobics experience more heart rate acceleration in simulated public speaking situations than do generalized social phobics, either in the same public speaking paradigm (Levin et al., submitted for publication) or in a simulated socialization challenge (Heimberg et al., 1990). The findings suggest that discrete social phobics experience prominent peripheral autonomic symptoms that are alleviated by beta blockers. Generalized social phobics, on the other hand, appear to experience less peripheral autonomic activation and more centrally mediated interpersonal hypersensitivity that seems highly responsive to MAOIs.

Benzodiazepines

There are no controlled studies of benzodiazepines in social phobia, but two open clinical trials of the triazolobenzodiazepine alprazolam suggest clinical efficacy. Lydiard et al. (1988) studied four patients with discrete and generalized social phobic features, all of whom benefited significantly from alprazolam in doses ranging from 2 to 8 mg/day. Interestingly, three of them had had prior tricyclic trials and failed to benefit substantially. One patient had had a further augmentation of response when phenelzine was added to the alprazolam. This patient was the only one with a childhood onset; he also had the longest-lasting condition and received the highest alprazolam dose of the four patients.

Reich and Yates (1988) entered 17 social phobics in an open eight-week trial with alprazolam; 14 completed the study. Of the 14, 11 had symptom reduction of 50 percent or greater. The only reported side effects of alprazolam in this dose range (1–7 mg/day, mean at week 8 of 2.9 mg/day) were sedation and disinhibition, which responded to a reduced dose.

The data suggest the efficacy of alprazolam, but controlled trials are needed to establish efficacy in comparison to placebo, as well as to other active drugs.

Other Medications

There are no placebo-controlled trials of a tricyclic antidepressant in a social phobic population. A number of investigators reported lack of efficacy in open trials, however, in patients who subsequently responded to phenelzine (Liebowitz et al., 1986), tranylcypromine (Versiani et al., 1988), or alprazolam (Lydiard et al., 1988). Imipramine was only of limited benefit in reducing interpersonal sensitivity in atypical depressives (Liebowitz et al., 1984) as well, suggesting limited utility in social phobia. In contrast to this is the reported efficacy of chlorimimpramine in comparison to diazepam in a mixed agoraphobic-socially phobic group for which the social phobic results are not reported separately (Allsopp et al., 1984). Also, Benca et al. (1986) reported imipramine to be helpful in two social phobics who also suffered from mitral valve prolapse. If controlled studies do not reveal the efficacy of tricyclics in social phobia, this would be an important difference from panic disorder and agoraphobia with panic attacks, which do respond well to tricyclics (Zitrin et al., 1983).

Goldstein (1987) has reported clonidine efficacy in a patient with social phobia characterized mainly by blushing who failed prior trials with benzodiazepines, phenelzine and propranolol.

Clinical Management

Once the diagnosis of social phobia is made, one should differentiate discrete performance anxiety from more generalized social phobia. The discrete social phobic who has difficulty with occasional speeches or perfor mances can be given a beta blocker such as propranolol to use as needed, such as an hour before the performance. The dosage has to be individualized, starting with 10–20 mg as a single dose and increasing it if necessary. Patients need to be advised that the heart rate should not drop below 55–60/minute; patients with low resting heart rates, such as highly conditioned athletes, may have difficulty using beta blockers.

Phenelzine is my preferred treatment at this time for patients with generalized social phobia, starting with 15–30 mg/day and building up. Patients need to follow a low-tyramine diet and avoid sympathomimetics. Side effects such as insomnia or postural hypotension can be treated if necessary.

Alprazolam may also have a role in social phobia, although at present I use it only adjunctively unless MAOIs are contraindicated. We are about to begin a buspirone study in social phobia. Group cognitive behavioral therapy (CGBT) as developed by Heimberg for social phobia (Heimberg et al., 1990) may be a useful alternative to or augmentation for pharmacotherapy, and a study is now underway to compare phenelzine and CGBT.

SIMPLE PHOBIAS

Definition

DSM III-R defines simple phobia as a persistent fear of a circumscribed stimulus (object or situation), excluding the fear of having a panic attack or of humiliation or embarrassment in social or performance situations. The response occurs almost invariably upon exposure to the feared stimulus, which is therefore routinely avoided or endured with dread. The fear or avoidant behavior has to be of sufficient magnitude to interfere significantly with normal daily routines, activities, or relationships, or there has to be marked distress about the fear, which the affected individual recognizes as excessive and unreasonable.

General Aspects

A number of recent books on anxiety disorders contain excellent overviews of simple phobia (Fyer, 1987; Marks, 1987; Barlow, 1988) to which the reader is referred. The remainder of this chapter will focus on recent findings about simple phobia concerning psychopharmacological management.

Psychopharmacological Treatment

Very little psychopharmacological research has been attempted with simple phobic individuals. Although numerous in the general population, according to epidemiological surveys (Myers et al., 1984), such patients usually do not come to psychiatric research facilities seeking treatment. This may be due to an absence of severe disability in most simple phobias and/ or to the patients' amenability to behavioral treatment techniques. Also, there exists a prevailing clinical view, without empirical support, that simple phobias are not helped by psychopharmacological treatment. As illustrated below, from a theoretical point of view, as well as from the few studies that have been reported, this belief does not seem justified.

Findings with Theoretical Implications for the Pharmacotherapy Response

Cameron et al. (1986) compared the symptom profiles of 316 anxiety disorder patients with a variety of diagnoses, including 142 with simple phobias. They found simple phobics to differ from social phobics and panic disorder patients in having less anxiety and phobic anxiety, and less fear of going crazy, losing control, or dying. Simple phobics did report comparable degrees of tachycardia, however.

This study suggests similar autonomic arousal but less emotional arousal in simple phobics compared to other phobic groups. Several other investigations have compared simple phobics and social phobics on autonomic arousal. Johansson and Lars-Goran (1982) placed socially phobic and claustrophobic individuals in social and confined situations while measuring heart rate. Both groups showed increases over baseline while in their feared situation, but increases were greater among the socially phobic individuals in the social simulation. This finding contrasts with the earlier one of Weerts and Lang (1978), who found that analogue subjects who feared spiders showed greater heart rate increases on imaginal exposure to these feared stimuli than did similarly recruited individuals who feared public speaking. Ohman (1986) also reported greater heart rate activation in animal phobics than in social phobics on exposure to slides of people engaging in the subjects' feared activity. These data suggesting heart rate activation in simple phobics raise the possibility of therapy with beta blockers.

In terms of emotional arousal, McNally and Steketee (1985) surveyed 22 patients seeking treatment for animal phobias to determine what they believed would happen if they encountered the feared object. Of the 22, 41 percent feared being attacked by the object, 18 percent feared going insane from fright, 14 percent feared being embarrassed if others noticed their fear, 14 percent feared accidental injury while fleeing in a panic, and 9 percent having a heart attack from fright. As the investigators noted, a majority feared harm not so much from the feared animal as from their own intense emotional reaction, suggesting that tranquilizers such as benzodiazepines might be of some benefit, at least during the initial stages of exposure. As discussed below, existing empirical data support this notion.

Curtis's group (Himle et al., 1989) have suggested subdividing simple phobia into four subtypes based on the particular fear: animal (including insect) fears; situational fears, including heights, closed spaces, etc; fear of choking; and blood injury phobia. Supporting these distinctions are subtype differences in age of onset, family history, frequency of associated spontaneous anxiety episodes, etc. In particular, Himle et al. suggest that situational phobics are more closely related to panic disorder patients with agoraphobia. Situational phobics often have as a single fear the same situations (planes, elevators, etc.) that agoraphobics also avoid. In addition, situational phobics lead the other simple phobic groups in reported unprecipitated anxiety episodes suggestive of panic attacks, and also have an older age of onset (in their twenties), more similar to panic disorder and agoraphobia. These observations suggest that some situational phobics might respond to the treatments found useful for panic disorder with and without agoraphobia, such as triazolobenzodiazepines (Sheehan et al., 1980), tricyclics (Zitrin et al., 1983), or MAOIs (Sheehan et al., 1980).

We have used medication to treat several patients with flying phobia who became panicky on airplanes but did not suffer panic attacks in any other situation. With acute alprazolam administration, these patients were able to fly after years of avoidance.

Marks (1988) recently reviewed blood injury phobia. He noted the distinctive biphasic autonomic arousal pattern characterized by initial tachycardia followed by substantial bradycardia. This parasympathetic response causes the characteristic symptoms of syncope and nausea. No pharmacological treatment has been reported, but benzodiazepines prior to planned exposure like blood drawing might be helpful, especially for blood injury phobics who are so fearful that they avoid medical care.

Psychopharmacological Studies in Simple Phobia

Zitrin et al. (1983) had a simple phobic comparison group that did not respond to imipramine preferentially over placebo in their agoraphobia trials. Retrospectively, however, (Fyer 1987) was able to identify a subgroup of simple phobics who experienced recurrent limited-symptom attacks (characterized by autonomic arousal, light-headedness, unsteadiness, or abdominal distress) in what came to be phobic situations and who did show benefit from imipramine (Fyer, 1987). An example given is a man who feared and avoided only bridges; his illness reportedly began when he felt nauseous and light-headed once while driving across a bridge.

Bernadt et al. (1980) studied drug plus exposure therapy in 22 snake or spider phobic volunteers. One and one-half hours before exposure, the subjects were given a single dose of either tolamolol (a beta blocker) 200 mg, diazepam 10 mg, or placebo. The beta blocker reduced the heart rate on exposure, while the benzodiazepine increased subjects' ability to approach their feared object. Neither medication did much for subjective fear, however.

An earlier study looked at the effect of different diazepam regimens on exposure therapy outcome in simple phobics. Marks (1972) randomly assigned 18 patients to two-hour sessions of live exposure in a partial crossover design that compared the effects of four drug regimens: exposure 1 hour after oral diazepam 0.1 mg/kg (peak diazepam); exposure four hours after the same dose (waning diazepam); or exposure one or four hours after placebo. Phobias improved under all four conditions, but more so with waning diazepam than placebo, with peak diazepam in between.

CONCLUSIONS

The role for pharmacotherapy in simple phobia remains to be determined. As is true for social phobia, the above-cited literature for simple phobia suggests that future psychopharmacological studies of simple phobia should focus on diagnostic and, to the extent that they can be identified, pathophysiological subtypes. The specificity of medications to different subtypes could help elucidate the relationships of these disorders to other anxiety disorders, and could also characterize the heterogeneity within simple phobia.

REFERENCES

Aimes PL, Gelder M, Shaw PM: Social phobia: A comparative clinical study. *Br J Psychiatry* 142:174–179, 1983.

Allsopp L, Cooper GL, Poole PH: Clomipramine and diazepam in the treatment of agoraphobia and social phobia in general practice. *Curr Med Res Opinion* 9(1):64–70, 1984.

Barlow D: *Anxiety and Its Disorders*. New York, Guilford Press, 1988.

Benca R, Matuzas W, Al-Sadir J: Social phobia, MVP, and response to imipramine. *J Clin Psychopharmacol* 6(1):50–51, 1986.

Bernadt M, Silverstone T, Singleton W: Behavioural and subjective effects of beta-adrenergic blockade in phobic subjects. *Br J Psychiatry* 137:452–457, 1980.

Bryant B, et al: Social difficulty in a student sample. *Br J Ed Psychol* 44:13–21, 1974.

Cameron O, Thyer BA, Nesse RM, et al: Symptom profiles of patients with DSM-III anxiety disorders. *Am J Psychiatry* 143(9):1132–1137, 1986.

Deltito J, Perugi G: A case of social phobia with avoidant personality disorder treated with MAOI. *Compr Psychiatry* 27(3):255–258, 1986.

Falloon I, Lloyd GG, Harpin RE: Real-life rehearsal with non-professional therapists. *J Nerv Ment Dis* 169:180–184, 1981.

Fyer AJ: Agoraphobia, in Klein D. (ed): *Anxiety*. New York, Karger, 1987, pp 91–126.

Goldstein S: Treatment of social phobia with clonidine. *Biol Psychiatry* 22:369–372, 1987.

Gorman J, Liebowitz MR, Fyer AJ, et al: Treatment of social phobia with atenolol. *J Clin Psychopharmacol* 5:298–301, 1985.

Heimberg RG, Becker RE, Goldfinger BA, et al: Treatment of social phobia by exposure, cognitive restructuring, and homework assignments. *J Nerv Ment Dis* 173(4):236–245, 1985.

Heimberg RG, Hope D, Dodge CS, et al: DSM III subtypes of social phobia: Comparison of generalized social phobias and public speaking phobics. *J Ment Ner Dis* 178:172–179, 1990.

Himle J, McFee K, Cameron OG, et al: Simple phobia: Evidence for heterogeneity. *Psychiatry Res* 28:25–30, 1989.

Johansson J, O. Lars-Goran: Perception of autonomic reactions and actual heart rate in phobic patients. *J Behav Assessment* 4(2):133–143, 1982.

Liebowitz M, Fyer AJ, Gorman JM, et al: Phenelzine in social phobia. *J Clin Psychopharmacol* 6(2):93–98, 1986.

Liebowitz M, Gorman JM, Fyer AJ, et al: Social phobia: Review of a neglected anxiety disorder. *Arch Gen Psychiatry* 42:729–736, 1985.

Liebowitz M, Gorman JM, Fyer AJ, et al: Pharmacotherapy of social phobia: An interim report of a placebo-controlled comparison of phenelzine and atenolol. *J Clin Psychiatry* 49(7):252–257, 1988b.

Liebowitz M, Quitkin FM, Stewart JW, et al: Antidepressant specificity in atypical depression. *Arch Gen Psychiatry* 45:129–137, 1988a.

Liebowitz MR, Quitkin FM, Stewart JW, et al: Phenelzine versus imipramine in atypical depression. *Arch Gen Psychiatry* 41:669–677, 1984.

Lydiard R, Larana MT, Howell EF, et al: Alprazolam in the treatment of social phobia. *J Clin Psychiatry* 49(1):17–19, 1988.

Marks IM: Enhanced relief of phobias by flooding during waning diazepam effect. *Br J Psychiatry* 121:493–505, 1972.

Marks IM: *Fears, Phobias, and Rituals*. New York, Oxford University Press, 1987.

Marks IM: Blood-injury phobia: A review. *Am J Psychiatry* 145(10):1207–1213, 1988.

Marks IM, Gelder MG: Different ages of onset in varieties of phobia. *Am J Psychiatry* 123:218–221, 1966.

McNally R, Steketee GS: The etiology and maintenance of severe animal phobias. *Behav Res* 23(4):431–435, 1985.

Mullaney J, Trippett CJ: Alcohol dependence and phobias: Clinical description and relevance. *Br J Psychiatry* 135:563–573, 1979.

Myers J, Weissman MM, Tischler G, et al: Six-month prevalence of psychiatric disorders in three communities: 1980–1982. *Arch Gen Psychiatry* 41:959–967, 1984.

Ohman A: Face the beast and fear the face: Animal and social fears as prototypes for evolutionary analyses of emotion. *Psychophysiology,* 23(2):123–145, 1986.

Pollard CA, Henderson J: Four types of social phobia in a community sample. *J Nerv Ment Dis* 176(7):440–445, 1988.

Reich J, Yates W: A pilot of treatment of social phobia with alprazolam. *Am J Psychiatry* 145(5):590–594, 1988.

Sheehan D, Ballenger J, Jacobson G: Treatment of endogenous anxiety with phobic and hypochondriacal symptoms. *Arch Gen Psychiatry* 37:51–59, 1980.

Smail P, Stockwell T, Canter S, et al: Alcohol dependence and phobia anxiety states. I. A prevalance study. *Br J Psychiatry* 144:53–57, 1984.

Thyer B, Parrish RT, Curtis GC, et al: Ages of onset of DSM-III anxiety disorders. *Comp Psychiatry* 26(2):113–122, 1985.

Turner S, Beidel DC, Dancu CV, et al: Psychopathology of social phobia and comparison to avoidant personality disorder. *J Abnorm Psychol* 95(4):389–394, 1986.

Versiani M, Klein DF, Nardi AE, et al: Tranylcypromine in social phobia. *J Clin Psychopharmacol* 8:279–283, 1988.

Weerts T, Lang PJ: Psychophysiology of fear imagery: Differences between focal phobia and social performance anxiety. *J Consult Clin Psychol* 46(5):1157–1159, 1978.

Zitrin C, Klein DF, Woerner MG, et al: Treatment of phobias. *Arch Gen Psychiatry* 40:125–138, 1983.

6

Clinical Management of
Generalized Anxiety Disorder

RUDOLF HOEHN-SARIC AND DANIEL R. MCLEOD

Generalized anxiety disorder (GAD), as defined in DSM III (American Psychiatric Association, 1980) and redefined in DSM III-R (American Psychiatric Association, 1987), represents a "residual" entity, consisting of persistent anxiety without the panic attacks, phobias, etc., that define other anxiety disorders. For generalized anxiety to be diagnosed, it must be experienced independently of symptoms that define other anxiety disorders. The main features of GAD are the presence of psychic symptoms, including unrealistic or excessive anxiety and worry, which should bother the person more often than not for at least six months, and somatic symptoms, such as increased muscular tension, autonomic hyperactivity, and hyperarousal. The diagnosis of GAD cannot be made if anxiety is part of other disorders frequently associated with increased anxiety, such as mood disorders, psychotic disorders, or specific organic conditions such as hyperthyroidism.

Clinically, GAD is not the sharply delineated disorder that DSM III-R makes it appear to be. Phenomenologically, GAD is closer to normal anxiety than are other anxiety disorders, and the border between normal and pathological anxiety is not sharp. In this context, it is of interest to observe that animal models identify only anxiolytics that are effective in GAD, not medications that relieve symptoms specific to other anxiety disorders, such as panic attacks (File et al., 1985). Thus, GAD may be an exaggerated form of a normal biological response common to both humans and animals. GAD may exist as a disorder by itself, but it may also precede (Cloninger et al., 1981; Hoehn-Saric and Barksdale, 1983; Garvey et al., 1988), accompany (Barlow, 1985), or follow (Katon et al., 1987) the onset of other anxiety disorders. It is frequently present in depression (Barlow, 1985), and GAD may interact with the symptoms of another anxiety disorder. For example, it may exacerbate obsessive-compulsive symptoms (Marks, 1987), but it may also have a life of its own. In the latter case, it can persist or even increase in intensity after the symptoms of another disorder, such as attacks of panic disorder, have been successfully treated (Waddell et al., 1984). Thus, GAD needs to be viewed as a therapeutic challenge in its own right, whether it occurs alone or in combination with other disorders.

THE ROLE OF PSYCHOLOGICAL TREATMENT IN GAD

Management of GAD patients almost always requires psychological intervention and frequently, but not invariably, pharmacotherapy. Psychological interventions consist of assurance, explanation of somatic symptoms, clarification of conflicts, and, if necessary, more complex therapeutic intervention to help the patient acquire coping mechanisms through reorganization of maladaptive attitudes, acquisition of new skills, and changes in life style (Frank et al., 1978).

Numerous studies have shown that psychological interventions are helpful in anxiety disorders (Freedman, 1980). However, there is little evidence suggesting that specific techniques yield better results in the treatment of GAD than basic psychotherapeutic interactions common to all psychological interventions (Frank et al., 1978). Improvement has been noted even with minimal contact, such as the administration of placebo (Banner and Meadows, 1983), connective tissue massage (McKechnie et al., 1983), physical exercise (Morgan, 1979), a pilgrimage to Lourdes (Morris, 1982), counseling by general practitioners (Catalan et al., 1984), various relaxation and meditation techniques (Shader and Greenblatt, 1983), temperature and muscle activity feedback (Banner and Meadows, 1983), nondirective psychotherapy (Blowers et al., 1987; Borkovec and Mathews, 1988), cognitive/behavior therapy techniques (Blowers et al., 1987; Borkovec and Mathews, 1988), and specifically targeted anxiety management training (Hutchings et al., 1980). Some studies suggest that, when combined, relaxation and a cognitive approach yield better results than either technique alone (Hutchings et al., 1980; Woodward and Jones, 1980). However, one has to keep in mind that the subjects in studies range from anxious college students to groups of poorly described anxious outpatients, and only a few studies have examined clearly defined GAD patients. Many studies are also flawed by methodological problems that make interpretation of the results difficult. Moreover, they deal with group data and artificial time limits rather than concentrating on the needs of the individual.

INTERACTIONS BETWEEN PSYCHOTHERAPY AND PHARMACOTHERAPY

Since the time when anxiolytic medications were introduced, many therapists have expressed concern that medications would interfere with treatment by lowering the patient's motivation to explore psychic problems or cooperate in behavioral tasks. Thus, they believe that medications may impede the acquisition of new coping skills and place the patient at a disadvantage once drug therapy is discontinued.

At present, there are no well-controlled studies examining interactions between medications and psychological treatments in GAD patients. However, studies using patients with other anxiety disorders or mixed groups consisting of predominantly anxious outpatients suggest that a combination of psychotherapy and pharmacotherapy does not hinder, but actually enhances, the outcome of therapy (Luborsky et al., 1975). Behavior therapy may also be favorably influenced by medication. Mavissakalian (1988) reported that the effects of exposure and imipramine were mutually potentiating in the treatment of agoraphobics, and Marks et al. (1972) found diazepam, particularly in the weaning phase, to be helpful in the flooding treatment of phobias.

Medication, however, may be counterproductive when its effects fail to match a patient's expectations. Hafner and Milton (1977) exposed agoraphobic patients, who were premedicated with propranolol or placebo, to feared situations and found placebo to be superior. They concluded that during several hours of exposure, propranolol gradually lost its effectiveness, resulting in an increased heart rate in the patients. This signaled an increase in anxiety to them as exposure progressed. The opposite, namely, a gradual decrease of an initially rapid heart rate, occurred in patients on placebo congruent with a decrease in anxiety during exposure.

Drug therapy may have a negative effect on the maintenance of improvement after the discontinuation of treatment. Patients who have become used to the anxiety-reducing effects of medications may become less tolerant of the discomforts caused by anxiety than patients who have gone through drug-free psychological training and who have learned to accept certain levels of anxiety as a part of life. For instance, Fontaine et al. (1984) found that the sudden withdrawal of medication after four weeks of treatment caused more rebound anxiety in patients who had received benzodiazepines than in those who had received placebo. This reaction cannot be attributed to benzodiazepine withdrawal, since nonanxious volunteers who received therapeutic doses of diazepam over six weeks noticed no unpleasant effects after the sudden discontinuation of the drug (McLeod et al., 1988). In another study, patients who received diazepam were able to reduce, but not discontinue, the drug after they had received anxiety management training (Laughren et al., 1986).

The anxiety-reducing effects of drug therapy may reduce therapists' efforts to improve patients' coping style and decrease patients' motivation for self-improvement. For example, patients with chronic free-floating anxiety who received electromyographic (EMG) feedback alone practiced relaxation exercises more frequently and maintained higher levels of improvement during follow-up than patients who had received diazepam (Lavallée et al., 1977). Reviewing the evidence from various studies, Marks (1982) concluded that phobic and obsessive-compulsive patients treated with behavior therapy maintained their improvement longer than those treated with drugs.

The maintenance of improvement after discontinuation of treatment may depend less on the use of medication during treatment than on therapist and patient expectancies regarding therapy, as well as the personality traits of the patients. This is illustrated in a study by Frank et al. (1978), who compared two groups of nonpsychotic outpatients receiving the same therapeutic intervention, except for the emphasis placed on self-help in one group and on medication in the other group. Actually, both groups received placebo and were seen in regular sessions in which they had to perform certain tasks. One group was told that the medication would improve their symptoms and that the tasks were being used to measure the progress of drug therapy (medication group). The other group was told that medication would be of some help, but that the crucial part of therapy was the acquisition of new skills through practice on tasks that would eventually be helpful in the management of real-life situations (mastery group). Over nine weeks of treatment, both groups improved to the same extent, but at a follow-up examination three months later, only the mastery group had maintained its improvement. Frank et al. (1978) further divided patients into a group with an internal locus of control (i.e., the general expectancy that events are contingent upon one's own behavior and, therefore, are under personal control) and a second group with an external locus of control (i.e., the belief that events are unrelated to one's own behavior and are primarily a matter of luck, fate, chance, or some powerful outside agent) (Rotter, 1966). Internally oriented patients improved significantly more in the mastery than in the medication condition. The opposite was true for external patients. Thus, regardless of the pharmacological action of a drug, patient and therapist expectancies and patients' personality traits may have a powerful influence on the long-term outcome of pharmacotherapy in nonpsychotic patients.

MEDICATIONS USED IN THE TREATMENT OF GAD

Benzodiazepines

Benzodiazepines, the most frequently prescribed drugs in GAD, are more often obtained from family physicians than from psychiatrists (Beardsley et al., 1988). Acting through the benzodiazepine–GABA receptor complex, a subsystem of the GABA system, benzodiazepines inhibit neuronal activity. They have widespread effects on the brain that manifest themselves through sedation, muscle relaxation, anxiety reduction, and an increased seizure threshold (Tallman et al., 1980). In addition, benzodiazepines lower sympathetic tone, not only through central mechanisms, but through direct action on the peripheral sympathetic ganglia (Surai and Costa, 1973) and the adrenal medulla (Kataoka et al., 1984) as well. The most pronounced effects of benzodiazepines are on vigilance and somatic anxiety. Benzodiazepines lower hypervigilance, inducing relaxation and, at higher doses, somnolence. In contrast to other anxiety-reducing medications, benzodiazepines not only reduce somatic symptoms, that is, the subjectively experienced bodily sensations such as increased muscle tension, palpitations, increased perspiration, or hyperactivity of the gastrointestinal tract, but also produce favorable alterations in physiological states. Acute administration of benzodiazepines leads to a lowering of skin conductance and a measure of sympathetic tone, and prevents the rise of blood pressure seen during stressful experimental sessions (Hoehn-Saric and McLeod, 1986; McLeod et al., 1988). Clinical doses of alprazolam also lower blood epinephrine levels (Stratton and Halter, 1985; Hoehn-Saric et al., 1986). The muscle-relaxing effects of benzodiazepines are well known but, on objective measures, they are weak and transitory (Lossius et al., 1980). In clinical doses, they are probably related more to a decrease in general arousal than to a direct effect on the muscular system.

In contrast to hypervigilance and somatic manifestations, psychic symptoms are less affected by benzodiazepines (Rickels, 1978; Hoehn-Saric et al., 1988). Even when regularly administered benzodiazepines only slightly decrease a person's tendency to worry, to ruminate, or to be hypersensitive in interpersonal relationships.

The anxiolytic effectiveness of benzodiazepines when given over a short period of time is well documented (for reviews, see Freedman, 1980; Shader and Greenblatt, 1983; Beckmann and Haas, 1984). Whether they maintain their effectiveness during long-term use, however, is less clear. In placebo-controlled studies, the differences between active medication and placebo decrease over time, which may be due to the development of tolerance to benzodiazepines or to the improvement of patients in the placebo group. Tolerance to the sedative (McLeod et al., 1988), anticonvulsant (Gonsalves and Gallager, 1987), and muscle-relaxant (Lossius et al., 1980) properties of benzodiazepines occurs when they are taken regularly. However, we did not observe the development of tolerance to autonomic effects when diazepam (McLeod, et al., 1988) or alprazolam (Hoehn-Saric et al., 1986) was administered in clinical doses over a six-week period. It is unknown whether tolerance develops to the anxiolytic properties of benzodiazepines. Animal data suggest that such tolerance does not develop (Lippa et al., 1977) or, if it does, it occurs much later than other forms of tolerance (Vellucci and File, 1979). In humans, tolerance to the anxiolytic effects of benzodiazepines can be observed in some patients, but most continue to benefit from them without a dose increase (Hollister, 1977; Uhlenhuth et al., 1988).

A large number of benzodiazepines are available to the clinician (see Table 6–1). Except for alprazolam, which also has antidepressant properties (Dawson et al., 1984), benzodiazepines do not differ pharmacodynamically. However, they do differ in their speed of absorption in the

Table 6–1 Benzodiazepines

	Drug Names		Active Metabolites	Half-Life Including Metabolites (Hr)	Rate of Absorption
	Generic	*Trade*			
Long-acting (T½ = >24 hr)	Chlordiazepoxide	Librium	+	36–200	Intermittent
	Diazepam	Valium	+	20–100	Rapid
	Clorazepate	Tranxene	+	36–200	Rapid
	Prazepam	Centrax	+	36–200	Intermittent
	Flurazepam	Dalmane	+	40–250	Rapid
Intermediate- to short-acting (T½ = 5–24 hr)	Alprazolam	Xanax		6–20	Intermittent
	Lorazepam	Ativan		10–20	Intermittent
	Temazepam	Restoril		8–22	Variable-Slow
	Oxazepam	Serax		4–15	Variable-Slow
Ultra-short acting (T½ = 1.5–5 hr)	Triazolam	Halcion		1.5–5	Intermittent

brain and in their half-lives (Greenblatt et al., 1981). Quickly absorbed drugs, such as diazepam, are useful for fast relief from anxiety, but they have a greater addiction potential than those with slower absorption rates (Griffiths et al., 1984). Benzodiazepines with long half-lives are advantageous when regular administration is indicated, but they may accumulate in patients with slow clearance, particularly in the elderly and in patients with liver disease (Hoyumpa, 1978; Salzman et al., 1983). Orientals also tend to have a lower clearance for benzodiazepines (Lin et al., 1988). Plasma levels of benzodiazepines correspond roughly to the oral dose. However, they vary considerably among patients and are poorly related to clinical effects and psychomotor performance (McLeod et al., 1988). Therefore, blood levels are generally not of clinical value.

The main side effect of benzodiazepines is sedation. The sedative effect of a single dose decreases with regular use. Long-acting benzodiazepines, however, may accumulate in the body and cause increased drowsiness even after prolonged use (McLeod et al., 1988). However, one has to keep in mind that drowsiness is not always caused by medication but may be the result of insomnia. In such cases, drowsiness improves when benzodiazepines restore sleep (Fabre et al., 1984). Mild cognitive and memory impairments can be demonstrated even in persons who take benzodiazepines in clinical doses (McLeod et al., 1988), but these impairments are not serious, except in persons with great sensitivity to benzodiazepines and in the elderly (Pomara et al., 1984). Increased anger, dysphoria, and disinhibition of suppressed behavior have been observed with benzodiazepines (Rosenbaum et al., 1984; Wilkinson, 1985). These effects appear mainly in persons with a predisposition to such behavior. Whether the regular use of benzodiazepines over prolonged periods of time causes brain damage remains unclear. Three computed tomography (CT) scan studies suggest a relationship between prolonged benzodiazepine use and the enlargement of cerebral ventricles (Lader et al., 1984; Schmauss and Krieg, 1987; Uhde and Kellner, 1987), while another study found no such relationship (Poser et al., 1983). Petursson et al. (1983) reported diminished psychomotor functioning in chronic benzodiazepine abusers. However, Lucki et al. (1985), who examined persons who had taken benzodiazepines for five years, found their patients' psychomotor function to be comparable to that of a nonmedicated control group.

Benzodiazepines are compatible with most medications. They enhance the effects of alcohol and sedatives. Cimetidine increases blood levels of benzodiazepines (Desmond et al., 1980), but such drug interactions usually are not of clinical significance.

The greatest drawback of benzodiazepines is their addiction potential, which, while lower than that of barbiturates, is nonetheless present (Marks, 1983). Fortunately, most patients take less benzodiazepine medication than prescribed and reduce their use over time. The pattern of abuse, namely, the gradual increase over time, is rare and is generally associated with multiple-drug abuse (Woods et al., 1988). Benzodiazepines that have a fast absorption rate, such as diazepam, create in the individual a sense of feeling "high" and are therefore more addictive than benzodiazepines with slower absorption rates (Griffiths et al., 1984). On the other hand, dependency, that is, difficulty in decreasing a therapeutic dose, can develop in patients using medications within a therapeutic range. Noyes et al. (1988) reported that withdrawal symptoms developed in nearly one-half of the patients who used benzodiazepines for more than a year. The severity of withdrawal symptoms depends on the dose, the length of use, and the patient's personality. Patients with a history of substance abuse are more prone to become dependent on benzodiazepines (Ciraulo et al., 1988). Benzodiazepine withdrawal symptoms resemble anxiety symptoms, making it difficult to know whether patients who decrease or discontinue benzodiazepines experience the reemergence of drug-suppressed anxiety, experience withdrawal symptoms, or both. Withdrawal symptoms consist of persistent anxiety, insomnia, irritability, dysphoria, and poor concentration. In more severe cases, patients may experience perceptual hypersensitivity, paresthesias, muscle pain and weakness, and, rarely, epileptic fits or schizophreniform psychosis (MacKinnon, 1982; Noyes et al., 1988; Soyka et al., 1988). A gradual lowering of the benzodiazepine dose generally makes withdrawal tolerable, although patients taking higher doses experience more severe withdrawal symptoms than those taking lower doses (Soyka et al., 1988). Since withdrawal symptoms vanish within two weeks, it is possible to assess the actual anxiety levels in patients within three or four weeks after the decrease or discontinuation of medication.

In summary, benzodiazepines are very versatile drugs that can be taken in a single dose or on a regular basis. Their beneficial effect on hyperarousal and the autonomic nervous system renders them particularly useful in the treatment of anxiety associated with somatic manifestations. Their main disadvantage is their addiction potential, which can be reduced considerably when benzodiazepines are taken on a regular basis only for a short time or, when possible, on an as-needed basis. Reviewing the evidence, Uhlenhuth et al. (1988) concluded that the risks of overuse, dependence, and addiction with benzodiazepines are low in relation to the massive exposure to benzodiazepines in our society. Many patients continue to derive benefits from long-term treatment with benzodiazepines, and opposition to the use of these drugs may be depriving many anxious patients of appropriate treatment.

Antidepressants

The effectiveness of antidepressants in treating panic attacks is well documented (Sheehan et al., 1980). Until recently, it was assumed that antidepressants were ineffective in or actually excerbated GAD (Klein, 1981) unless depression coexisted. Several reviews of the effect of tricyclic antidepressants (Liebowitz et al., 1988) in mixed anxiety depressive states have found antidepressants to be equal or even superior to benzodiazepines. Only in one study were benzodiazepines superior to antidepressants. A recent study by Kahn et al. (1986) examined 242 anxiety neurotic patients, many of whom fell into the diagnostic category of GAD. Results of the study demonstrated that imipramine, a tricyclic antidepressant, was more effective than chlordiazepoxide in reducing anxiety. During the first two weeks the benzodiazepine was superior, but after the second week, the effect of imipramine began to exceed that of chlordiazepoxide. Both drugs were, however, superior to placebo.

Hoehn-Saric et al. (1988) recently compared the benzodiazepine alprazolam with the antidepressant imipramine in a group of 60 patients who had a DSM-III-R diagnosis of GAD and no history of previous panic attacks. When the anxiolytic effects were measured with scales that combined psychic and somatic items, alprazolam was more effective than imipramine during the first week, but in subsequent weeks both drugs appeared to be equal. However, when psychic and somatic scales were examined separately, it was found that imipramine affected predominantly the psychic symptoms of anxiety. Patients reported that they worried and ruminated less, felt less dysphoric, and experienced less discomfort in interpersonal relationships. These effects were not seen after a single dose of imipramine but gradually appeared after two or more weeks on medication. Vigilance was reduced in some patients, for whom imipramine induced drowsiness, but was heightened in those for whom it produced increased excitability and insomnia. This hyperalertness tended to decrease over a period of several weeks.

The effect of imipramine on somatic symptoms was complex. Symptoms associated with sympathetic arousal, such as palpitations and increased perspiration, either were not affected or were exacerbated during the first week of medication. In some patients these symptoms persisted indefinitely, but in most patients they decreased gradually. After four weeks of treatment, they reached levels comparable to those seen in patients treated with benzodiazepines. Objective evidence, however, contradicted the subjective reports. Imipramine increased the heart rate and the systolic blood pressure not only after the initial dose of 25 mg, but after six weeks on medication as well, in spite of patients' subjective reports that cardiac symptoms had decreased during that period. There are at least two explanations for the discrepancies between subjective improvement and the objective findings. It is possible that the improvement in psychic symptoms leads to a disregard of bodily cues, and thus to an apparent improvement in cardiac symptoms. The other possibility is that imipramine exercises a stabilizing effect on the sympathetic manifestations of anxiety through its effect on the locus coeruleus-noradrenergic system, and patients perceive this stabilization as improvement (Hoehn-Saric et al., 1981; Nutt, 1989). Gastrointestinal symptoms often improve with imipramine, possibly due to its anticholinergic activity. Imipramine has no direct effect on the muscular system.

Only imipramine has been studied in selected GAD patients. Studies of mixed populations, however, suggest that other tricyclic antidepressants, as well as mianserin (Khan et al., 1983) and trazodone (Wheatley, 1976), may have anxiolytic effects. The mechanism of action of antidepressants in GAD is not clear. Tricyclic antidepressants block the reuptake of norepinephrine and serotonin in the synaptic cleft. Since activation of the central noradrenergic system is associated with anxiety, it has been postulated that imipramine-induced increases in norepinephrine at the sites of the alpha-2 autoreceptors inhibit the activity of the noradrenergic system and subsequently decrease the level of anxiety (Redmond and Huang, 1979). We observed that inhibition of the noradrenergic system with the selective alpha-2 agonist clonidine lowered anxiety, but we were more impressed by its stabilizing effect on fluctuations in anxiety (Hoehn-Saric et al., 1981). Thus, it appears that the noradrenergic system serves as an amplification system for anxiety, and antidepressants may have a stabilizing effect resulting in a reduction of fluctuations in anxiety.

The serotonergic system has also been associated with the psychobiology of anxiety. Kahn et al. (1988) suggested that anxiety occurs when the serotonergic system is oversensitized. Medications that block serotonin reuptake gradually desensitize the oversensitive serotonin receptor, thus reducing anxiety. This theory, however, is not supported by animal data (Blier et al., 1988). At present, one can only say that the serotonergic and noradrenergic systems are somehow involved in the regulation of anxiety. The mechanisms are not yet sufficiently understood, and since the effects of antidepressants appear only after two weeks, they probably involve secondary adaptive mechanisms.

Many antidepressants, including imipramine, also have antihistaminic and anticholinergic properties. The sedating antihistaminic effect contributes to the anxiolytic effects, whereas the anticholinergic effects may have a beneficial effect on gastrointestinal hypermotility but usually cause undesirable side effects. Side effects of imipramine occur as the consequence of increased sympathetic tone and anticholinergic activity. They may seriously interfere with the therapeutic effects of imipramine and may make it impossible at times to increase the dose to a therapeutic level. Feelings of tension, agitation, insomnia, palpitations, orthostatic hypotension, perspiration, dry mouth, difficulty urinating, and constipation are frequent. Very disturbing erectile or ejaculatory impotence may occur in men. Imipramine also has quinidine-like effects on the heart's conductivity and can be cardiotoxic (Risch et al., 1982). Therefore, it should be administered with caution in persons who have cardiac illnesses. Anticholinergic effects also may cause cognitive impairment and confusion in susceptible individuals. Drowsiness due to antihistaminic effects occurs in some persons. Caution should be exercised when imipramine is combined either with medications that have sympathomimetic or anticholinergic properties or with monoamine oxidase inhibitors.

In summary, the candidate for treatment with imipramine is the GAD patient who experiences excessive chronic worrying. The onset of the anxiolytic action of imipramine is gradual, beginning only during the second week of regular treatment. The effectiveness of imipramine tends to increase over subsequent weeks (Kahn et al., 1986; Hoehn-Saric et al., 1988). Since anxiety patients are preoccupied with bodily sensations, they are sensitive to the side effects of medications. Therefore, it is advisable to start with small doses in order to avoid premature dropout and to increase the medication gradually. In our experience, the average effective dose of imipramine is lower than that needed for the treatment of depression (Hoehn-Saric et al., 1988). Sedation or sympathetic arousal, when present, diminishes gradually, but anticholinergic effects tend to persist. In spite of general improvement, some patients continue to suffer from insomnia and experience somatic symptoms when stressed. In such patients, the addition of a benzodiazepine is useful. Tolerance to the anxiolytic effects of imipramine does not develop, and there is no abuse potential. Since other antidepressants have fewer side effects, it is important to examine them systematically for their anxiolytic properties.

BUSPIRONE

Buspirone, an azaspirodecanedione, is an anxiolytic that is structurally and pharmacologically unrelated to benzodiazepines. Other drugs with similar mechanisms are under investigation. Buspirone binds as an agonist to the serotonin 1A receptor, which is probably an autoreceptor (Eison and Temple, 1986). Since the activation of this receptor inhibits serotonergic activity, it is possible that the anxiolytic effects of buspirone are linked to a decrease of serotonergic action in the brain. Gepirone (Csanalosi et al., 1987), a close analogue with similar properties, and ritanserin (Ceulemans et al., 1985), a postsynaptic serotonin-2-receptor antagonist, also have been reported to decrease anxiety. Interestingly, buspirone increases rather than decreases the activity of the noradrenergic locus coeruleus (Sanghera et al., 1983), which suggests that some dimensions of anxiety can be reduced in spite of stimulation of the noradrenergic system.

Buspirone appears to decrease symptoms associated with cognitive and interpersonal problems. Patients appear less concerned about anger, hostility, and interpersonal attention (Rickels et al., 1982). Vigilance and hyperalertness are not affected, except by large doses (Goa and Ward, 1986). Buspirone decreases somatic symptoms, but to a lesser degree than benzodiazepines (Rickels et al., 1982). The pharmacological profile of buspirone shows no indication that the drug, given in clinical doses, has a direct effect on the autonomic or muscular systems (Goa and Ward, 1986).

The side effects of buspirone are mild and consist primarily of drowsiness, nausea, and headaches. Buspirone appears to be compatible with most medications, and it does not potentiate the effects of alcohol or sedatives (Goa and Ward, 1986). There is no evidence of tolerance or addiction potential for buspirone. Buspirone shows no cross-tolerance to benzodiazepines and is not useful in the treatment of benzodiazepine withdrawal symptoms (Goa and Ward, 1986).

An individual dose of buspirone has only a weak anxiolytic action. The drug has to be taken regularly for two weeks or more to be fully effective (Goa and Ward, 1986). Thus, buspirone is not helpful to the patient who needs immediate relief from anxiety. It is more effective in patients who have not taken benzodiazepines previously, since those who have tend to miss the immediate relaxing and mellowing effects of benzodiazepines. As with imipramine, its use is indicated in persons who suffer predominantly from chronic psychic anxiety and need regular medication. In our experience, a mixture of buspirone with benzodiazepines can be advantageous in patients with high levels of both psychic and somatic anxiety.

ANTIHISTAMINES

Antihistamines block histamine-1 receptors in the brain. Since the histamine system contributes to wakefulness, antihistamines induce drowsiness and sedation (Schwartz, 1979). Antihistamines also block cholinergic receptors, and this gives them anticholinergic properties as well (Rickels et al., 1970).

Antihistamines have weak anxiolytic effects that surpass those of placebo only at doses that produce marked side effects (Rickels et al., 1970). Their effects on anxiety have been investigated less extensively than those of other medications used in GAD. It appears, however, that antihistamines have little effect on psychic anxiety.

Antihistamines decrease vigilance and hyperalertness and are sedating. Their effects on autonomic nervous system are mixed. Because of their anticholinergic properties, antihistamines can increase the heart rate, and they may potentiate the sedative and atropine-like effects of other drugs (Rickels et al., 1970). However, they also decrease gastrointestinal activity. They have no direct effect on the muscular system. Mild tolerance to the sedative effects may occur with chronic use. However, the drugs appear to have no addiction potential.

Because of their quick action, antihistamines can be administered in single doses or as a regular prescription. In spite of their weak anxiolytic action, they remain popular because they are not habit-forming and can be given safely to persons who are likely to abuse medications.

BETA-ADRENERGIC BLOCKERS

As is evident from their name, beta-adrenergic blockers neutralize the effects of epinephrine and norepinephrine on the beta receptors. Some but not all beta blockers cross the blood-brain barrier (Noyes, 1985). In clinical doses, however, the anxiolytic effects of all beta blockers are peripheral rather than central (Tyrer, 1976). Their main effect is a slowing of the heart rate, which decreases the perception of physical distress in anxiety-provoking situations.

Beta blockers have no direct effect on psychic anxiety and do not affect vigilance or hyperalertness (Tyrer, 1976). They reduce the cardiac response to anxiety by decreasing heart rate and lowering blood pressure. Beta blockers may increase the peristalsis of the gastrointestinal tract, thereby exaggerating rather than diminishing the effects of anxiety on this system. On the other hand, they reduce tremor, which may enhance the patient's self-confidence. Beta blockers lower fluctuations of cardiac, but not of psychic or other autonomic, manifestations of anxiety.

In large doses, those beta blockers that cross the blood-brain barrier may cause tiredness, vivid dreams, depression, and, rarely, delirium (Noyes, 1985). Caution is necessary when combining beta blockers with medications that lower blood pressure, and they should be avoided in patients with bradycardia, heart block, cardiac failure, asthma, or bronchospasm. Rebound hypertension may occur in hypertensive patients in whom beta blockers are suddenly withdrawn. Neither tolerance nor addiction occurs with them (Noyes, 1985).

In summary, beta blockers are useful in the treatment of patients with palpitations or irregular heartbeat. The attenuation of the cardiac response may have a calming effect in some patients. Beta blockers have a rapid clinical effect and can be taken either in single doses or on a regular schedule. When other distressing anxiety symptoms coexist, it is advantageous to combine beta blockers with a benzodiazepine.

NEUROLEPTICS

A number of neuroleptics, including loxapine, trifluoperazine, thioridazine, and others, have demonstrated some anxiolytic properties (Chou and Sussman, 1988). Animal studies have shown that the dopaminergic system is involved in stress responses (Hoehn-Saric, 1982) and it is probable that the dopamine receptor–blocking properties of neuroleptics reduce anxiety. Some neuroleptics have antihistaminic properties, which cause sedation, and this may be of additional benefit. While prescribed frequently in the past, particularly in persons with substance abuse potential, neuroleptics are rarely used in treating anxiety disorders today because of their tendency to cause tardive dyskinesia. Neuroleptics should be reserved for the rare patient with GAD who seems to respond selectively to such drugs.

MANAGEMENT OF THE GAD PATIENT

The description of GAD in DSM III-R fails to convey the variability and complexity of the disorder. Each case has to be considered individually according to the severity and chronicity of the disorder, the somatic symptoms, the presence of environmental stressors, and specific personality traits. In the majority of cases, GAD is a chronic condition, but the severity of symptoms may depend greatly on the degree of stress currently present. Patients may exhibit subclinical anxiety during periods of low stress and the full picture of GAD during times of increased pressure. Some patients experience high anxiety during certain times, for example, in the morning when facing a difficult work situation, but only low anxiety on weekends or during vacation. Other patients are sensitive to any unexpected change and focus their anxieties on internal events, such as unusual body sensations, or on external events, such as the lateness of a spouse in coming home from work. Such patients constantly anticipate some disaster. Only rarely do patients complain about general tension deprived of content.

Not only psychic but also somatic symptoms vary greatly in GAD. Some patients experience predominantly cardiac symptoms, while others complain mostly of gastrointestinal or muscular symptoms (Hoehn-Saric et al., 1989). The level of hyperarousal also varies. Most patients complain of insomnia, but some patients have less difficulty sleeping or suffer from only occasional periods of insomnia.

Finally, one has to consider the interaction of heightened anxiety with patients' personality traits. GAD may lead to overconscientiousness in some patients but to histrionic outbursts in others. Type A patients may make aggressive attempts to cope with anxiety-provoking situations, while passive type B patients may react with fearful withdrawal. Patients with a strong need for control prefer learning better coping techniques to taking medication; the opposite is true for passive, dependent persons with an external locus of control (Frank et al., 1978).

In the management of the patient with GAD, one must first exclude possible organic causes for the condition. Since many patients are concerned about their health, they appreciate a thorough medical workup and a detailed explanation of the results. Patients should also be encouraged to abstain from caffeine-containing beverages (Lee et al., 1985) and excessive use of alcohol.

Mild forms of anxiety generally respond well to simple psychological interventions (Catalan et al., 1984) and usually do not require medication, except perhaps for an occasional pill for better sleep or to aid in the management of specific stressful situations. Benzodiazepines as well as anti-histamines are useful in such conditions, since they have a rapid onset of action and can be taken when needed.

In more severe forms of GAD, it becomes necessary to see the patient regularly and to provide psychological help. Depending upon the patient's adjustment, this help may range from simple counseling and relaxation techniques to specific anxiety management approaches or intensive psychotherapy.

Most patients with severe anxiety also need medication to lower their anxiety levels. Table 6–2 provides an overview of the medication given in GAD. For reduction of general tension, hyperalertness, insomnia, and other physical symptoms, benzodiazepines are the most effective drugs. Benzodiazepines should be given on a regular basis for several weeks to provide steady relief. During this time, one should help patients master coping techniques. An exception is the patient who is at high risk for substance abuse. In such a patient, antihistamines, although less effective than benzodiazepines, are the medications of choice. Some patients with a strong need for control prefer to take benzodiazepines only when they feel stressed rather than on a regular basis. Such requests should be respected.

As a regular prescription, benzodiazepines with longer half-lives are preferable because they have a more consistent effect than those with short half-lives. Benzodiazepines with short half-lives have to be taken several times a day to prevent rebound anxiety. When given as a sedative, they may cause early morning insomnia (Kales et al., 1983). On the other hand, in the elderly or in patients with liver disease, a benzodiazepine with a shorter half-life should be chosen to avoid accumulation and excessive sedation. Benzodiazepines with fast absorption rates should be avoided when taken on a regular basis because they carry a higher risk of addiction.

Since benzodiazepines have a direct effect on the autonomic system and decrease muscle tension, they are useful in patients with somatic symptoms. In the presence of pronounced cardiac symptoms, high doses of benzodiazepines may be needed (Hoehn-Saric and McLeod, 1987). In such cases, the addition of a beta blocker can reduce the dose of benzodiazepine required.

An important question is how long a patient should remain on a regular regimen of benzodiazepines. Several studies have shown that benzodiazepines tend to maintain their anxiolytic effectiveness even when given over prolonged periods (Uhlenhuth et al., 1988). However, Rickels et al. (1986) found that of 131 patients in whom treatment was discontinued after a six-month diazepam maintenance study, 37 percent were still symptom free one year later. Most patients who relapsed did so within three months, and 67 percent stated that their symptoms interfered significantly with their lives. These data showed that the majority of patients need long-term or intermittent support or medication. However, a sub-

Table 6–2 Effects of Anxiolytic Medication: An Overview

	Benzodiazepines	Imipramine	Buspirone	Antihistamines	Beta Blockers
Anxiolytic effects					
Apprehension	↓ ↓ ↓	↓ ↓ ↓	↓ ↓	↓ ↓	0
Vigilance	↓ ↓ ↓	(↑ ↓)	(↓)	↓ ↓	(↓)
Autonomic effect					
Subjective	↓ ↓ ↓	↓ ↓	↓ ↓	↓ ↑	↓ ↓ ↓
Objective	↓ ↓ ↓	↓ ↑	0	0	↓ ↓ ↓
Muscular effect	↓	0	0	0	0
Onset of action	Acute	Gradual	Gradual	Acute	Acute
Tolerance	Yes	No	No	No	No
Abuse potential	Yes	No	No	No	No

Note: ↓ = decrease; ↑ = increase; 0 = no effect; parentheses indicate a weak effect.

stantial number of patients remain symptom free for a year. For such patients, a few weeks of benzodiazepine treatment seems to suffice. Therefore, attempts should be made every four to six weeks to reduce the dose. When benzodiazepines have been given for long periods, Rickels (personal communication) negotiates an agreement with patients to reduce the dose to the point of complete withdrawal, but promises to reinstitute medication should they continue to experience significant levels of anxiety four weeks after discontinuation. Most patients can be weaned completely or placed on medication on an as-needed basis. Only patients who experience constant, intense distress should be kept on or reinstated on a regular long-term medication program.

Patients with intense psychic symptoms may profit from buspirone or an antidepressant. The disadvantage of these medications is that they have no immediate effect and thus have to be taken regularly. While no controlled studies exist, clinical experience suggests that antidepressants are much more potent than buspirone. Since neither buspirone nor antidepressants lower autonomic activity, a combination of these drugs with a benzodiazepine may be useful in patients with situational exacerbation of somatic symptoms.

Regardless of the medication or the way in which it is prescribed, it remains important to tell the patient that a drug is a helpful adjuvant in the effort to acquire better coping mechanisms; it is not an end in itself. Patients should be constantly encouraged to reorganize their lives and develop better coping strategies that will permit them to live without medication or, if medication is necessary, with the lowest possible dose.

REFERENCES

American Psychiatric Association: *Diagnostic and Statistical Manual of Mental Disorders* (DSM III), ed 3. Washington, D.C.: American Psychiatric Association, 1980, pp 232–233.

American Psychiatric Association: *Diagnostic and Statistical Manual of Mental Disorders,* ed 3, rev. Washington, D.C.: American Psychiatric Association, 1987, pp 251–253.

Banner CN, Meadows WM: Examination of the effectiveness of various treatment techniques for reducing tension. *Br J Clin Psychol* 22:183–193, 1983.

Barlow DH: The dimensions of anxiety disorders, in Tuma AH, Maser J (eds): *Anxiety and the Anxiety Disorders*. Hillsdale, NJ: Lawrence Erlbaum, 1985, pp 479–500.

Beardsley RS, Gardocki GJ, Larson DB, et al: Prescribing of psychotropic medication by primary care physicians and psychiatrists. *Arch Gen Psychiatry* 45:1117–1119, 1988.

Beckmann H, Haas S: Therapie mit Benzodiazepinen: Eine Bilanz. *Nervenarzt* 55:111–121, 1984.

Blier P, de Montigny C, Chaput Y: Electrophysiological assessment of the effects of antidepressant treatments on the efficacy of 5-HT neurotransmission. *Clin Neuropharmacol* 11(suppl 2):1–10, 1988.

Blowers C, Cobb J, Mathews A: Generalized anxiety: A controlled treatment study. *Behav Res Ther* 25:493–502, 1987.

Borkovec TD, Mathews AM: Treatment of nonphobic anxiety disorders: A comparison of nondirective, cognitive, and coping desensitization therapy. *J Consult Clin Psychol* 56:877–884, 1988.

Catalan J, Gath D, Edmonds G, et al: The effects of nonprescribing of anxiolytics in general practice I. Controlled evaluation of psychiatric and social outcome. *Br J Psychiatry* 144:593–602, 1984.

Ceulemans D, Hoppenbruwers ML, Gelders Y, et al: The effects of benzodiazepine withdrawal on the therapeutic efficacy of a serotonin antagonist in anxiety disorder. *Abstracts: 4th World Congress of Biological Psychiatry,* Philadelphia, September 8–13, 1985, p 58.

Chou JCY, Sussman N: Neuroleptics in anxiety. *Psychiatr Ann* 18:172–175, 1988.

Ciraulo DA, Sands BF, Shader RI: Critical review of liability for benzodiazepine abuse among alcoholics. *Am J Psychiatry* 145:1501–1506, 1988.

Cloninger CR, Martin RL, Clayton P, et al: A blind follow-up and family study of anxiety neurosis: Preliminary analysis of the St. Louis 500, in Klein DF, Rabkin JG (eds): *Anxiety: New Research and Changing Concepts.* New York, Raven Press, 1981, pp 137–154.

Csanalosi I, Schweizer E, Case WG, et al: Gepirone in anxiety: A pilot study. *J Clin Psychopharmacol* 7:31–33, 1987.

Dawson GW, Jue SG, Brogden RN: Alprazolam: A review of its pharmacodynamic properties and efficacy in the treatment of anxiety and depression. *Drugs* 27:132–147, 1984.

Desmond PV, Patwardhan RV, Schenker S, et al: Cimetidine impairs elimination of chlordiazepoxide (Librium) in man. *Ann Intern Med* 93:266–268, 1980.

Eison AS, Temple DL Jr: Buspirone: Review of its pharmacology and current perspectives on its mechanisms of action. *Am J Med* 80(suppl 38):1–9, 1986.

Fabre LF, Johnson PA, Greenblatt DJ: Drowsiness sedation levels in anxious neurotic outpatients. *Psychopharmacol Bull* 20:128–136, 1984.

File SE, Pellow S, Chopin P: Can animal tests of anxiety detect anti-panic compounds? *Abstract: Society for Neuroscience,* Vol. II, Part 2. Fifteenth annual meeting, Dallas, Texas, October 20–25, 1985, p 273.

Fontaine R, Chouinard G, Annable L: Rebound anxiety in anxious patients after abrupt withdrawal of benzodiazepine treatment. *Am J Psychiatry* 141:848–852, 1984.

Frank JD, Hoehn-Saric R, Imber SD, et al: *Effective Ingredients of Successful Psychotherapy.* New York, Brunner-Mazel, 1978.

Freedman AM: Psychopharmacology and psychotherapy in the treatment of anxiety. *Pharmacopsychiatry* 13:277–289, 1980.

Garvey MJ, Cook B, Noyes R Jr: The occurrence of a prodrome of generalized anxiety in panic disorders. *Compr Psychiatry* 29:445–449, 1988.

Goa KL, Ward A: Buspirone: A preliminary review of its pharmacological properties and therapeutic efficacy as an anxiolytic. *Drugs* 32:114–129, 1986.

Gonsalves SF, Gallager DW: Time course for development of anticonvulsant tolerance and GABA-ergic subsensitivity after chronic diazepam. *Brain Res* 405:94–99, 1987.

Greenblatt DJ, Shader RI, Divoll M, et al: Benzodiazepines: A summary of pharmacokinetic properties. *Br J Clin Pharmacol* 11:11S–16S, 1981.

Griffiths RR, McLeod DR, Bigelow GE, et al: Comparison of diazepam and oxazepam: Preference, liking and extent of abuse. *J Pharmacol Exp Ther* 229:501–508, 1984.

Hafner J, Milton F: The influence of propranolol on the exposure in vivo of agoraphobics. *Psychol Med* 7:419–425, 1977.

Hoehn-Saric R: Neurotransmitters in anxiety. *Arch Gen Psychiatry* 39:735–742, 1982.

Hoehn-Saric R, Barksdale VC: Impulsiveness in obsessive-compulsive patients. *Br J Psychiatry* 143:177–182, 1983.

Hoehn-Saric R, McLeod DR: Physiological and performance responses to diazepam: Two type of effects. *Psychopharmacol Bull* 22:439–443, 1986.

Hoehn-Saric R, McLeod DR: Cardiac symptoms and anxiety disorders: Contributing factors and pharmacological treatment. *Am J Cardiol* 60:68J–73J, 1987.

Hoehn-Saric R, McLeod DR, Zimmerli WD: Differential effects of alprazolam and imipramine in generalized anxiety. Presented at the 15th Collegium Internationale Neuro-Psychopharmacologicum Congress, San Juan, Puerto Rico, December 14–17, 1986.

Hoehn-Saric R, McLeod DR, Zimmerli WD: Differential effects of alprazolam and imipramine in generalized anxiety. *J Clin Psychiatry* 49:293–301, 1988.

Hoehn-Saric R, McLeod DR, Zimmerli WD: Differences in symptom presentation and treatment response among anxious patients with high versus low levels of cardiac complaints. *Am J Psychiatry* 146:854–859, 1989.

Hoehn-Saric R, Merchant A, Keyser M, et al: Effects of clonidine on anxiety disorders. *Arch Gen Psychiatry* 38:1278–1282, 1981.

Hollister LE: Valium: A discussion of current issues. *Psychosomatics* 18:45–58, 1977.

Hoyumpa AM: Disposition and elimination of minor tranquilizers in the aged and in patients with liver disease. *South Med J* 71(suppl 2):23–28, 1978.

Hutchings DF, Denney DR, Basgall J, et al: Anxiety management and applied relaxation in reducing general anxiety. *Behav Res Ther* 18:181–190, 1980.

Kahn RJ, McNair DM, Lipman RS, et al: Imipramine and chlordiazepoxide in depressive and anxiety disorders: II. Efficacy in anxious outpatients. *Arch Gen Psychiatry* 43:79–85, 1986.

Kahn RS, van Praag HM, Wetzler S, et al: Serotonin and anxiety revisited. *Biol Psychiatry* 23:189–208, 1988.

Kales A, Soldatos CR, Bixler EO, et al: Early morning insomnia with rapidly eliminated benzodiazepines. *Science* 220:95–97, 1983.

Kataoka Y, Gutman Y, Guidotti A, et al: Intrinsic GABA-ergic system of adrenal chromaffin cells. *Proc Natl Acad Sci USA* 18:3218–3222, 1984.

Katon W, Vitaliano PP, Anderson K, et al: Panic disorder: Residual symptoms after the acute attacks abate. *Compr Psychiatry* 28:151–158, 1987.

Khan MC, Bennie EH, Stulemeijer SM, et al: Mianserin and doxepin in the treatment of outpatients depression with anxiety. *Br J Clin Pharmacol* 15:213S–218S, 1983.

Klein DF: Anxiety reconceptualized, in Klein DF, Rabkin JG, (eds): *Anxiety: New Research and Changing Concepts*. New York, Raven Press, 1981, pp 235–263.

Lader MH, Ron M, Petursson H: Computed axial brain tomography in long-term benzodiazepines users. *Psychol Med* 14:203–206, 1984.

Laughren TP, Dias AM, Keene C, et al: Can chronically anxious patients learn to cope without medications? *McLean Hosp J* 11:72–77, 1986.

Lavallée YJ, Lamontagne Y, Pinard G, et al: Effects on EMG feedback, diazepam and their combination on chronic anxiety. *J Psychosom Res* 21:65–71, 1977.

Lee MA, Cameron OG, Greden JF: Anxiety and caffeine consumption in people with anxiety disorders. *Psychiatry Res* 15:211–217, 1985.

Liebowitz MR, Fyer AJ, Gorman JM, et al: Tricyclic therapy of the DSM-III anxiety disorders: A review with implication for further research. *J Psychiatr Res* 22(suppl 1):7–31, 1988.

Lin KM, Lau JK, Smith R, et al: Comparison of alprazolam plasma levels in normal Asian and Caucasian male volunteers. *Psychopharmacology* 96:365–369, 1988.

Lippa AS, Greenblatt EN, Pelham RW: The use of animal models for delineating the mechanism of action of anxiolytic agents, in Hanin I, Usdin E (eds): *Animal Models in Psychiatry and Neurology*. New York, Pergamon Press, 1977, pp 279–292.

Lossius R, Dietrichson P, Lunde PKM: Effect of diazepam and desmethyldiazepam in spasticity and rigidity. *Acta Neurol Scand* 61:378–383, 1980.

Luborsky L, Singer B, Luborsky L: Comparative studies of psychotherapies. Is it true that "everyone has won and all must have prizes". *Arch Gen Psychiatry* 32:995–1008, 1975.

Lucki I, Rickels K, Geller AM: Psychomotor performance following the long-term use of benzodiazepines. *Psychopharmacol Bull* 21:93–96, 1985.

MacKinnon GL: Benzodiazepine withdrawal syndrome: A literature review and evaluation. *Am J Drugs Alcohol* 9:19–39, 1982.

Marks I: Are there anticompulsive or antiphobic drugs? Review of the evidence. *Psychopharmacol Bull* 18:78–84, 1982.

Marks IM: *Fears, Phobias, and Rituals*. New York, Oxford University Press, 1987, p 433.

Marks IM, Viswanathan R, Lipsedge MS, et al: Enhanced relief of phobias by flooding during waning diazepam effects. *Br J Psychiatry* 121:493–505, 1972.

Marks J: The benzodiazepines—for good or evil. *Neuropsychobiology* 10:115–126, 1983.

Mavissakalian M: The mutual potentiating effects of imipramine and exposure in agoraphobia, in Hand I, Wittchen HV (eds): *Panic and Phobias*. Berlin, Springer-Verlag, 1988, pp 36–43.

McKechnie AA, Wilson F, Watson N, et al: Anxiety states: A preliminary report on the value of connective tissue massage. *J Psychosom Res* 27:125–129, 1983.

McLeod DR, Hoehn-Saric R, Labib AS, et al: Six weeks of diazepam treatment in normal women: Effects on psychomotor performance and psychophysiology. *J Clin Psychopharmacol* 8:83–99, 1988.

Morgan WP: Anxiety reduction following acute physical activity. *Psychiatr Ann* 9:36–45, 1979.

Morris PA: The effect of pilgrimage on anxiety, depression and religious attitude. *Psychol Med* 12:291–294, 1982.

Noyes R Jr: Beta-adrenergic blocking drugs in anxiety and stress, in Curtis CG, Thyer BA, Rainey JM (eds): *Psychiatric Clinics of North America: Anxiety Disorders*. Philadelphia, WB Saunders, 1985, pp 119–132.

Noyes R Jr, Garvey MJ, Cook BL, et al: Benzodiazepine withdrawal: A review of the evidence. *J Clin Psychiatry* 49:382–389, 1988.

Nutt DJ: Altered central alpha-2-adrenoreceptor sensitivity in panic disorder. *Arch Gen Psychiatry* 46:165–169, 1989.

Petursson H, Gudjonsson GH, Lader MW: Psychomotor performance during withdrawal from long-term benzodiazepine treatment. *Psychopharmacology* 81:345–347, 1983.

Pomara N, Stanley B, Block R, et al: Diazepam impairs performance in normal elderly subjects. *Psychopharmacol Bull* 20:137–139, 1984.

Poser W, Poser S, Roscher D, et al: Do benzodiazepines cause cerebral atrophy? *Lancet* 1:715, 1983.

Redmond DE Jr, Huang YH: New evidence for a locus coeruleus—norepinephrine connection with anxiety. *Life Sci* 25:2149–2162, 1979.

Rickels K: The use of antianxiety agents in anxious outpatients. *Psychopharmacology* 58:1–17, 1978.

Rickels K, Case WG, Downing RW, et al: One-year follow-up of anxious patients treated with diazepam. *J Clin Pharmacol* 6:32–36, 1986.

Rickels K, Gordon PE, Zamostien BB, et al: Hydroxyzine and chlordiazepoxide in anxious neurotic outpatients: A collaborative controlled study. *Compr Psychiatry* 11:457–474, 1970.

Rickels K, Wiseman K, Norstad N, et al: Buspirone and diazepam in anxiety: A controlled study. *J Clin Psychiatry* 43(sec 2):81–86, 1982.

Risch SC, Groom GP, Janowsky DS: The effects of psychotropic drugs on the cardiovascular system. *J Clin Psychiatry* 43(sec 2):16–31, 1982.

Rosenbaum JF, Woods SW, Groves JE, et al: Emergence of hostility during alprazolam treatment. *Am J Psychiatry* 141:792–793, 1984.

Rotter JB: Generalized expectancies for internal vs. external control of reinforcement. *Psychol Monogr* 80, No. 1 (whole no. 609), 1966.

Salzman C, Shader RI, Greenblatt DJ, et al: Long v short half-life benzodiazepines in the elderly. *Arch Gen Psychiatry* 40:293–297, 1983.

Sanghera MK, McMillan BA, German DC: Buspirone, a non-benzodiazepine anxiolytic, increases locus coeruleus activity. *Eur J Pharmacol* 86:107–110, 1983.

Schmauss C, Krieg JD: Enlargement of cerebrospinal fluid space in long-term benzodiazepine abusers. *Psychol Med* 17:869–873, 1987.

Schwartz JC: Histamine receptors in the brain. *Life Sci* 25:895–912, 1979.

Shader RI, Greenblatt DJ: Some current treatment options for symptoms of anxiety. *J Clin Psychiatry* 44(sec 2):21–29, 1983.

Sheehan DV, Ballenger J, Jacobson G: Treatment of endogenous anxiety with phobic, hysterical, and hypochondriacal symptoms. *Arch Gen Psychiatry* 37:51–59, 1980.

Soyka M, Steinberg R, Vollmer M: Entzugsphänomene bei schrittweisem Benzodiazepinentzug. *Nervenarzt* 59:744–748, 1988.

Stratton JR, Halter JB: Effect of a benzodiazepine (alprazolam) on plasma epinephrine and norepinephrine levels during exercise stress. *Am J Cardiol* 56:136–139, 1985.

Surai A, Costa E: Benzodiazepines and posttetanic potentiation in sympathetic ganglia of the bullfrog. *Brain Res* 50:235–239, 1973.

Tallman JH, Paul SM, Skolnick P: Receptors for the age of anxiety: Pharmacology of the benzodiazepines. *Science* 207:274–281, 1980.

Tyrer P: *The Role of Bodily Feelings in Anxiety*. London, Oxford University Press, 1976.

Uhde TW, Kellner CW: Cerebral ventricular size in panic disorder. *J Affective Disorders* 12:175–178, 1987.

Uhlenhuth EH, DeWit H, Balter MB, et al: Risks and benefits of long-term benzodiazepine use. *J Clin Psychopharmacol* 8:161–167, 1988.

Vellucci SV, File SE: Chlordiazepoxide loses its anxiolytic action with long-term treatment. *Psychopharmacology* 62:61–65, 1979.

Waddell MT, Barlow DH, O'Brien GT: A preliminary investigation of cognitive and relaxation treatment of panic disorder: Effects on intense anxiety vs "background" anxiety. *Behav Res Ther* 22:393–402, 1984.

Wheatley D: Evaluation of trazodone in the treatment of anxiety. *Curr Ther Res* 20:74–83, 1976.

Wilkinson CJ: Effects of diazepam (Valium) and trait anxiety on human physical aggression and emotional state. *J Behav Med* 8:101–114, 1985.

Woods JH, Katz JL, Winger G: Use and abuse of benzodiazepines: Issues relevant to prescribing. *JAMA* 260:3476–3480, 1988.

Woodward R, Jones RB: Cognitive restructuring treatment: A controlled trial with anxious patients. *Behav Res Ther* 18:401–401, 1980.

7

Obsessive-Compulsive Disorders: A Clinical Approach

MICHAEL A. JENIKE

OVERVIEW

Once considered a rare and refractory disorder, obsessive-compulsive disorder (OCD) is now recognized as a common illness that can be effectively treated in the majority of patients. Successful treatment usually consists of behavior therapy and psychotropic medication, which can be expected to improve the condition of most patients substantially, and occasionally completely, within a few months (Jenike et al., 1986).

Obsessions and compulsions of OCD can be severely incapacitating; not only are depression and anxiety frequently associated problems, but the symptoms often spread, interfering with functioning in almost all spheres of life and occasionally involving the person's family. We have seen several patients in our OCD clinic whose entire families were moved to a new house in an attempt to escape the patient's contamination fears and cleaning rituals.

DIAGNOSTIC CRITERIA

The currently accepted definition of OCD is given in the *Diagnostic and Statistical Manual of Mental Disorders-Revised* (DSM III-R) and states that a patient must have either obsessions or compulsions that are a significant source of distress to the individual or that interfere with social or role functioning. Obsessions are defined as "recurrent, persistent ideas, thoughts, images, or impulses that are ego-dystonic, i.e., they are not experienced as voluntarily produced, but rather as thoughts that invade consciousness and are experienced as senseless or repugnant. Attempts are made to ignore or suppress them." Compulsions are defined as "repetitive and seemingly purposeful behaviors that are performed according to certain rules or in a stereotyped fashion. The behavior is not an end in itself, but is designed to produce or prevent some future event or situation. However, either the activity is not connected in a realistic way with what it is designed to produce or prevent or it may be clearly excessive. The act is performed with a sense of subjective compulsion coupled with desire to resist the compulsion (at least initially). The individual generally recognizes the senselessness of the behavior (this may not be true for young children) and does not derive pleasure from carrying out the activity, although it provides a release of tension."

DISTINCTION FROM OBSESSIVE-COMPULSIVE PERSONALITY DISORDER

OCD is frequently confused with obsessive-compulsive personality disorder. OCD is an Axis I disorder in DSM III-R, while obsessive-compulsive personality disorder (Table 7–1) is an Axis II disorder. Although patients diagnosed with obsessive-compulsive personality disorder may have some obsessions and minor compulsions associated with their perfectionism, indecisiveness, or procrastination, these rituals do not interfere with the patient's life to the extent that OCD does. However, some patients with OCD also have compulsive personality traits, and some also meet DSM III-R criteria for obsessive-compulsive personality disorder (Rasmussen and Tsuang, 1986). Baer et al. (1989) found that only 6 percent of those patients who met the DSM-III criteria for OCD also met the criteria for DSM-III compulsive personality disorder using a standardized structured interview.

Table 7–1   DSM-III-R Criteria for Obsessive-Compulsive Personality Disorder

A pervasive pattern of perfectionism and inflexibility, beginning by early adulthood and present in a variety of contexts, as indicated by at least *five* of the following:

1. Perfectionism that interferes with task completion, e.g., inability to complete a project because the person's overly strict standards are not met
2. Preoccupation with details, rules, lists, order, organization, or schedules to the extent that the major point of the activity is lost
3. Unreasonable insistence that others submit to the person's way of doing things, or unreasonable reluctance to allow others to do things because of the conviction that they will not do them correctly
4. Excessive devotion to work and productivity, to the exclusion of leisure activities and friendships
5. Indecisiveness: decision making is either avoided, postponed, or protracted
6. Overconscientiousness, scrupulousness, and inflexibility about matters of morality, ethics, or values
7. Restricted expression of affection
8. Lack of generosity in giving time, money, or gifts when no personal gain is likely to result
9. Inability to discard worn-out or worthless objects even when they have no sentimental value

The differential diagnosis of these two disorders has important implications for treatment. For example, although traditional psychotherapy
produces little change in OCD obsessions and compulsions, it may be of
some value in the treatment of patients with obsessive-compulsive personality disorder (Jenike, 1986). Conversely, although behavior therapy
and psychopharmacological treatments have been found in controlled
trials to be very effective for OCD symptoms, there has been little research using these approaches for obsessive-compulsive personality disorder.

PREVALENCE

Although traditional estimates of the prevalence of OCD in the general
population were approximately 0.05 percent, recent studies have suggested a significantly higher lifetime prevalence of 2–3 percent (Meyers
et al., 1984; Robins et al., 1984); thus OCD is not the rare psychiatric
disorder it was once thought to be.

SUBTYPES OF OCD

Obsessive-compulsive symptoms tend to fall into several major categories: checking rituals, cleaning rituals, obsessive thoughts, obsessional
slowness, or mixed rituals. Checking and cleaning rituals form the overwhelming majority of compulsive rituals (53 and 48 percent, respectively)
(Hodgson and Rachman, 1977).

Cleaning Compulsions

A thirty-year-old male presented to our clinic with a fear of being contam-
inated by touching various objects he considered dirty. He had to cover
various "dirty" objects with paper towels before he was able to touch
them. If he did happen to touch his laundry, his bed, door handles in
public restrooms, his shoes, the gas cap on his car, or other "dirty" objects, he experienced vague feelings of dirtiness and discomfort, and he
engaged in extensive washing of his hands, along with any clothing that
he believed had come into contact with the object. The patient kept one
hand "clean" at all times and refused to place this hand in his trouser
pocket or to use it to shake hands. As a result of these OCD symptoms,
the patient was unable to work full time, and his social life dwindled.
(Note: Rachman and Hodgson, 1980, have noted similarities between patients with cleaning rituals and those with simple phobias. In both cases
a specific environmental situation triggers the fear, and the person en-
gages in passive avoidance of the situation or the contaminant, resulting
in a rapid decrease in anxiety.)

Checking Compulsions

A fifty-year-old female presented to our clinic who engaged in repetitive checking behaviors when she was not sure whether she had performed an action correctly. She plugged and unplugged electric appliances 20 times or more to be sure that she had actually taken the plug out of the socket. She did the same with light switches, turning them on and off repeatedly to ensure that she in fact had turned them off. She stared at the addresses on envelopes for up to several minutes to ensure that she had actually seen her name on the envelopes. She repetitively counted money, and her arithmetic required so many recalculations that she totally avoided financial paperwork and could no longer work in her previous job as a bookkeeper. The patient was no longer able to read because she continually returned to sentences she had already read to be sure that she had actually seen them.

Primary Obsessional Disorder

Virtually all patients with compulsive rituals also have frequent obsessive thoughts. However, there is a subgroup of OCD patients whose primary problem is obsessive thoughts, with few or no rituals present (Jenike et al., 1987a). These obsessive thoughts are typically of an aggressive, sexual, or religious nature and are repulsive to the sufferer. For example, a thirty-year-old male could no longer enter public places because of obsessive thoughts and impulses to shout obscenities or to accuse "unsavory" characters of having committed some illegal act. Similarly, a 32-year-old female no longer entered public places because she experienced intolerable sexual thoughts about individuals she saw in these places.

Other Types

Less common subtypes of OCD symptoms consist of rituals that involve placing objects in a certain order, and primary obsessional slowness, in which patients become "stuck" for hours while performing everyday tasks such as dressing and are unable to finish them. As larger numbers of OCD patients appear for treatment, relatively rare subtypes are being identified, such as patients with obsessions and compulsions aimed primarily at controlling an overwhelming fear of having a bowel movement or being incontinent of urine in public (Jenike et al., 1987b; Epstein and Jenike, 1990) or young women who have extensive face-picking rituals that can last for hours each day. Other disorders closely related to OCD are monosymptomatic hypochondriasis (Brotman and Jenike, 1984), dysmorphophobia (Jenike, 1984a), obsessive fear of AIDS (Jenike and Pato, 1986), cancer, or some other illness (Jenike, 1986a).

AGE OF ONSET OF OCD

There is a paucity of data on the age of onset of the major subtypes of OCD: patients with washing rituals alone, checking rituals alone, mixed rituals (washing, checking, repeating, or ordering), and obsessions in the absence of compulsions. DSM III-R (1987) does not relate subtypes to age of onset of OCD, stating that "although the disorder usually begins in adolescence or early adulthood, it may begin in childhood." Thyer et al. (1985) noted the lack of reliable data regarding age of onset for all anxiety disorders.

A search of the medical literature from 1966 to 1988 revealed several studies in which age of onset was reported for the general diagnosis of OCD but not for any particular subgroup. Black (1974) reported that the mean age of onset for OCD was in the early twenties, with over one-half of the patients becoming symptomatic by age 25 and three-quarters by age 30. Less than 5 percent had onset beyond 40 years of age. Rachman and Hodgson (1980), in a study of 83 patients with OCD, arrived at similar findings; 65 percent of the sample had onset prior to 25 years of age. Thyer et al. (1985) studied a group of 27 OCD patients and found a mean age of onset of 25.6 years. Rasmussen and Tsuang (1986) reported a mean age of onset in their 44 OCD patients of 19.8 years.

While establishing the mean age of onset of OCD in early adulthood, the earlier data provided little information concerning differences in age of onset among subtypes of OCD or between the sexes. A recent study of 138 consecutively evaluated OCD patients found significant differences in mean age of onset among subtypes (Minichiello et al., 1990). Patients with obsessions or cleaning rituals alone had comparable ages of onset (age 27), while those with checking rituals alone or mixed rituals had earlier onset (age 18–19) (Table 7–2). The finding of a significantly earlier age

Table 7–2 Mean Age of Onset (Years) of Subgroups of OCD Patients Based on Type of Ritual and Sex of Patient

Type of OCD	Sex of Patient		Total
	Male	Female	
Cleaners	21.8 ± 9.5	29.0 ± 13.5	27.2 ± 12.9
	n = 8	n = 25	n = 33
Checkers	14.4 ± 6.0	21.1 ± 13.4	18.1 ± 10.9
	n = 16	n = 19	n = 35
Mixed rituals	18.4 ± 8.5	20.1 ± 9.5	19.2 ± 8.8
	n = 25	n = 19	n = 44
Obsessions alone	25.6 ± 11.9	30.1 ± 14.7	27.0 ± 12.5
	n = 18	n = 8	n = 26
Total	19.8 ± 11.9	24.6 ± 11.9	22.3 ± 11.8
	n = 67	n = 71	n = 13

of onset for males (20 years) versus females (25 years) is consistent with the finding of a higher prevalence of childhood OCD in males (Flament and Rapoport, 1984).

PATIENTS WHO FAIL TO IMPROVE

Certain predictors of treatment failure have been identified, including noncompliance with treatment, concomitant severe depression (Foa, 1979), delusional beliefs in rituals or obsessions, presence of concomitant severe personality disorder (Jenike et al., 1986a, 1986b), and compulsive rituals. Patients with schizotypal and possibly other severe personality disorders (Axis II in DSM III-R) also do poorly (Jenike, 1986d; Minichiello et al., 1987; Baer et al., 1989).

Outcome studies and anecdotal evidence indicate that poor compliance with the behavioral treatment program is the most common reason for treatment failure with behavioral therapy for OCD (Marks, 1981). Behavior therapy is more demanding of the patient than many other forms of psychotherapy, and the patient must comply with behavioral instructions both during treatment sessions and during homework assignments. If the patient is inconsistent in doing this, treatment is unlikely to be successful. The aid of a family member or friend in carrying out homework assignments is often critical in ensuring compliance. In addition, the use of antidepressants concomitantly with behavioral therapy often increases patients' compliance with exposure treatments (Marks et al., 1980). New methods of improving compliance with behavioral treatment are under investigation, including the use of portable computers that assist the patient in carrying out homework assignments (Baer et al., 1987, 1989).

Severe depression has also been found to be a negative predictor for improvement with behavior therapy of OCD (Foa, 1979). In patients with severe depression (e.g., neurovegetative signs), the behavioral processes of physiological habituation to the feared stimuli do not occur, regardless of the length of exposure (Lader and Wing, 1969). Patients with severe depression often respond well to behavioral therapy procedures after their depression is controlled with medication (Baer and Minichiello, 1986).

If a patient has obsessive thoughts without rituals, behavioral therapy is unlikely to succeed. In these cases, pharmacotherapy is the treatment of choice.

Patients who strongly believe that their compulsive rituals are necessary to forestall future catastrophes (i.e., "overvalued ideas") appear to have a poorer outcome with behavioral treatments (Foa, 1979). For example, the patient who believes that someone in his family will die if he does not wash his entire house every day is unlikely to give up this ritual with behavior therapy alone. In some cases, treatment with antidepressant medication will produce changes in a patient's fixed beliefs, and behavior therapy may then be successful in eliminating rituals.

As noted above, patients who meet DSM III-R criteria for both OCD and schizotypal personality disorder do not respond well to either behavior therapy or pharmacotherapy. The idea of concomitant schizotypal personality disorder as a poor prognostic indicator in OCD appears to have validity in light of the literature on treatment failure. This personality disorder encompasses several of the poor predictive factors reviewed above. Most noticeably, these patients have a strong belief that their rituals are necessary to prevent some terrible event. Also, these patients have a difficult time complying with prescribed treatment and record-keeping tasks. Rachman and Hodgson (1980) have also found that the presence of an "abnormal personality" is a negative predictor of outcome in behavior therapy for OCD; more recently, Solyom et al. (1985) reported on a similar subcategory of patients with "obsessional psychosis," who also respond poorly to both behavior therapy and pharmacotherapy.

If a patient meets the criteria for schizotypal personality disorder, we attempt to arrange for placement in a structured environment such as a day treatment center or halfway house during and after behavioral treatment. This produces small decreases in obsessive and compulsive symptoms, along with moderate improvements in overall functioning.

Patients with contamination fears and cleaning rituals appear to respond best to behavioral treatment (Rachman and Hodgson, 1980), although those with checking compulsions may not respond as well. Even when they are responsive to behavioral techniques, patients with checking rituals appear to respond more slowly than those with cleaning rituals (Foa and Goldstein, 1978). A possible explanation for this difference is that many patients with checking rituals are unable to engage in the prescribed response prevention, especially those who check excessively at home (Rachman and Hodgson, 1980). In addition, patients with primary obsessional slowness respond more slowly to behavior therapy than do patients with either cleaning or checking rituals (Baer and Minichiello, 1986).

SOMATIC THERAPIES FOR OCD: DRUGS, ELECTROCONVULSIVE THERAPY, AND PSYCHOSURGERY

Drugs

Much has been learned about somatic treatments for OCD in the last few years. We now have medications that predictably help over one-half of these patients. The number of controlled trials is growing rapidly as OCD clinics are seeing large numbers of patients. The typical randomized, prospective, placebo-controlled trial, which proved so useful in depression research, had been almost impossible until recently because of the small number of OCD patients available to any one researcher. Anecdotal evidence and the few controlled trials that demonstrate the effectiveness of pharmacotherapy in some patients will be reviewed.

Heterocyclic Antidepressants

Numerous antidepressants have been reported to be useful in treating patients with OCD, including imipramine (Geissman and Kammerer, 1964; Hussain and Ahad, 1970; Angst and Theobald, 1980; Turner et al., 1980), amitriptyline (Hussain and Ahad, 1970; Snyder, 1980), doxepin (Ananth et al., 1975), desipramine (Gross et al., 1969), zimelidine (Kahn et al., 1984), fluoxetine (Fontaine and Chouinard, 1985), trazodone (Prasad, 1984; Lydiard, 1986), and fluvoxamine (Goodman et al., 1989). All of these reports, however, involved a small number of cases without any controls. Responses were unpredictable and not clearly related to depression; there was, however, dramatic improvement in some cases. Three recent controlled trials indicated that fluvoxamine was helpful in a number of OCD patients (Perse et al., 1987; Goodman et al., 1989; Jenike et al., 1990). In an open trial involving over 60 OCD patients, fluoxetine was effective in treating both OCD symptoms and depression (Jenike et al., 1989).

Clomipramine (Anafranil), a tricyclic antidepressant, has been available in Europe and Canada for over a decade, and anecdotal studies indicate that it may have some specific antiobsessional properties apart from its antidepressant qualities (Fernandez and Lopez-Ibor, 1967; De Vorvie, 1968; Grabowski, 1968; Jiminez, 1968; Lopez-Ibor, 1969; Marshall and Micev, 1973; Wyndowe et al., 1975; Yaryura-Tobias and Neziroglu, 1975; Yaryura-Tobias et al., 1976; Rack, 1977; Capstick, 1977; Waxman, 1977; Ananth et al., 1981; Coombe, 1982; Stroebel et al., 1984). A few carefully controlled studies have confirmed preliminary results that clomipramine is superior to placebo in the treatment of OCD (Ananth et al., 1979; Marks et al., 1980; Montgomery, 1980; Thoren et al., 1980a, 1980b; Insel et al., 1983; Jenike et al., 1989). A large, encouraging multicenter trial of clomipramine, funded by the Ciba-Geigy Pharmaceutical Company, has recently been completed in the United States (De Veaugh-Geiss et al., 1989), and clomipramine is now on the market. The main drawback to clomipramine is its occasionally troublesome side effects, which are primarily of an anticholinergic nature. Sexual difficulties are common, and there is a small incidence of seizures at higher doses. Many patients, however, tolerate it well.

Monoamine Oxidase Inhibitors

There are still no controlled studies on the use of monoamine oxidase inhibitors (MAOIs) in OCD. There exist a number of case reports (Joel, 1959; Annesley, 1969; Jain et al., 1970; Jenike, 1981; Rimher et al., 1982; Swinson, 1984), and anecdotal evidence suggests that they may be particularly helpful for patients who suffer concomitantly from OCD and panic attacks or severe anxiety (Jenike, 1982; Jenike et al., 1983). Affective illness in patients or their families does not appear to be a good predictor of responsiveness to MAOI (Jenike et al., 1983).

Lithium Carbonate

A link between manic-depressive illness and OCD has been suggested (Black, 1974; Stern and Jenike, 1983; Joseph Lipinski, personal communication, 1984). Cycling obsessive-compulsive symptoms have been described, but there are very few reports on the successful use of lithium carbonate in OCD. One double-blind crossover trial of six OCD patients carried out in Denmark reported that lithium was as ineffective as placebo in symptom resolution (Geisler and Schou, 1970). On the other hand, there are a few convincing case reports of classical OCD patients who improved with lithium carbonate (Forssman and Walinder, 1969; Van Putten and Sander, 1975; Stern and Jenike, 1983).

As mentioned earlier, obsessive-compulsive behaviors are sometimes found in patients suffering from bipolar affective disorder (Black, 1974; Baer et al., 1985). Although behavior therapy techniques of in vivo exposure and response prevention are highly effective in treating these behaviors (see the next section), until recently there were no reports of their use in patients with bipolar disorder and concomitant OCD. A recent report of two patients who met the criteria for both disorders, and who were treated with a combination of therapist-aided and self-administered exposure and response prevention, demonstrated that behavior therapy was effective only after their major affective disorder was controlled with lithium and neuroleptics (Baer et al., 1985).

Rasmussen (1984) reported a 22-year-old woman with classical OCD who did not respond to clomipramine alone but who improved greatly a few days after lithium carbonate was added, with a stabilized blood level of 0.9 mEq/L. Whether or not lithium augmentation of other tricyclic antidepressants or MAOIs for obsessive-compulsive symptoms is helpful remains to be tested. Improvement in depressives has been demonstrated in tricyclic nonresponders after addition of lithium to the antidepressant (De Montigny et al., 1981).

Antipsychotic Agents

Under stress, the severely obsessional patient may appear psychotic, an observation that prompted clinicians to attempt amelioration with neuroleptic drugs. Commonly, patients receive neuroleptics for many years, even though there is no evidence that they have been of any help.

There are only a few case reports of success with these agents (Altschuler, 1962; Hussain and Ahad, 1970; O'Regan, 1970a, 1970b; Rivers-Buckeley and Hollender, 1982). Most of these patients were atypical, and some presented the clinical picture of schizophrenia rather than classical OCD. It may be that the schizophrenic features were partly, or even substantially, responsible for the favorable outcomes.

In view of the absence of data on the efficacy of these agents and the frequency of toxic side effects, their use is recommended only for the more acutely disturbed obsessional patient. When these agents are tried, patients should be evaluated at regular intervals of not more than one month and the neuroleptic discontinued if there is no definite improvement.

Anxiolytic Agents

Once again, there are no good studies addressing the use of anxiolytics in patients with OCD. Most clinicians feel that these agents are of little use in the treatment of obsessions or compulsions but that they do decrease the anxiety that many OCD patients suffer. If antidepressants improve OCD, anxiety usually decreases without the use of anxiolytics.

The literature contains a few anecdotal reports of success (Breitner, 1960; Bethume, 1964; Hussain and Ahad, 1970; Tesar and Jenike, 1984; Tollefson, 1985) and a couple of controlled trials (Venkoba Rao, 1964; Orvin, 1967) where the outcome criteria were unclear. Buspirone was ineffective in a small open trial (Jenike and Baer, 1988).

In view of the occasional spontaneous remission and often fluctuating course of OCD, it is difficult to make a strong case for the use of anxiolytic drugs on the basis of available data.

Other Agents

Since a deficit in the brain's serotonergic system is sometimes hypothesized in patients with OCD, the use of the serotonin precursor tryptophan is of interest. Most of the work on tryptophan has been done by one group, and the results have not been replicated by others. Yaryura-Tobias and colleagues (1977, 1979, 1981) reported a number of patients who improved with tryptophan.

Rasmussen (1984) reported a male OCD patient who had a partial response to clomipramine that was dramatically boosted when 6 g/day of L-tryptophan was added. This patient relapsed when the tryptophan was stopped and improved again when it was restarted. Whether tryptophan can boost the antiobsessional effects of other tricyclic antidepressants or MAOIs remains to be determined. Walinder and associates (1976), however, demonstrated that L-tryptophan potentiates the effects of tricyclic antidepressant in endogenously depressed patients.

Since the administration of tryptophan stimulates the enzyme that causes the breakdown of tryptophan, to be maximally effective, nicotinamide and probably vitamins B_6 and C should also be administered. It is also likely that the administration of other large neutral amino acids should also be controlled in the diet and not taken in close proximity to doses of tryptophan (Cole et al., 1980; Jenike et al., 1986c).

Electroconvulsive Therapy

Since patients with OCD are refractory to the usual treatments, many receive courses of electroconvulsive therapy (ECT). Over one-third of the severe OCD patients who have been referred by clinicians to our OCD clinic during the past few years have had at least one course of ECT. Most did not suffer from a major affective disorder, and the main reason for administering ECT was for treatment of the OCD.

ECT is generally regarded as ineffective in the OCD patient who is not endogenously depressed (Gruber, 1971; *APA Task Force Report No. 14,* 1978), although scant literature exists concerning the effects of ECT alone on OCD. In a review of this subject, Mellman and Gorman (1984) found a few studies reporting that ECT in combination with other treatment modalities was associated with clinical improvement in some OCD patients. They also reported one atypical patient (obsessions alone, which developed after his wife's death) who had a good response to ECT after failing to respond to a number of treatments, including a twelve-week trial of clomipramine. Walter et al. (1972) assessed the combined effects of ECT, modified narcosis, and antidepressants on obsessional neurotics (unclear diagnostic criteria) and found that 40 percent of the patients improved. The relative effect of each form of treatment separately was obscure. Grimshaw (1965) studied 100 patients with obsessional symptoms, which were also poorly defined, and concluded that ECT had little effect on obsessional states.

Psychosurgery

Since most OCD patients who undergo psychosurgery have very severe illness that has not responded to multiple therapeutic approaches, the results of surgical intervention are impressive (Le Beau, 1952; Whitty and Duffield, 1952; Birley, 1964; Sykes and Tredgold, 1964; Strom-Olsen and Carlisle, 1971; Tan et al., 1971; Kelly et al., 1972; Bridges et al., 1974; Bailey et al., 1975; Bernstein et al., 1975; Mitchell-Heggs et al., 1976; Smith et al., 1976; Tippen and Henn, 1982; Jenike et al., 1986c; Ballantine et al., 1987).

Tippen and Henn (1982) reviewed the results of six studies of modified leukotomy that included 110 patients with obsessional disease. Nearly 81 percent (*n* = 89) were at least improved, and more than one-half of that group were in complete remission. The long-term outcome of these patients remains undetermined.

Side effects of modern site-specific lesion techniques are rare. The data on the efficacy of surgical treatment for OCD should be interpreted with some caution, however, since negative results are rarely reported. It is still unclear which OCD patients should be referred for surgical procedures, and definite recommendations must await further data.

BEHAVIOR THERAPY FOR OCD

Description

Behavior therapy is a directive psychotherapeutic approach, based on proven learning principles, that teaches patients how to alter directly their compulsive rituals. The techniques most consistently effective in reducing compulsive behaviors (and obsessive thoughts) are *exposure* to the feared situation or object and *response prevention,* in which the patient is helped to resist the urge to perform the compulsive act after this exposure.

Behavior therapy produces the largest changes in rituals, such as compulsive cleaning or checking, whereas changes in obsessive thoughts are less predictable (Marks, 1981). This is in contrast to the results of traditional psychotherapy, where the changes produced are mainly in obsessional thoughts, with little effect on rituals (Sturgis and Meyer, 1980). This difference reflects the specific effects of behavioral treatment, where the behaviors themselves are the targets of treatment. Consequently, behavior therapy is now regarded as an effective treatment when behavioral rituals predominate (Marks, 1981).

History of Behavioral Treatments for OCD

The use of behavioral techniques to treat obsessions and compulsions is not new. A century ago, Janet gave a remarkably accurate description of what is now termed "exposure therapy," including the name itself:

> The guide, the therapist, will specify to the patient the action as precisely as possible. He will analyze it into its elements if it should be necessary to give the patient's mind an immediate and proximate aim. By continually repeating the order to perform the action, that is, exposure, he will help the patient greatly by words of encouragement at every sign of success, however insignificant, for encouragement will make the patient realize these little successes and will stimulate him with the hopes aroused by glimpses of greater successes in the future. Other patients need strictures and even threats and one patient told [Janet], "Unless I am continually being forced to do things that need a great deal of effort I shall never get better. You must keep a strict hand over me." (Cited by Marks, 1981)

This outline of the behavioral treatment of OCD remains concise and accurate today, and exposure therapy as described by Janet remains the major behavioral treatment of OCD almost a century later. Yet despite the fact that behavioral techniques were successfully employed a century or more ago, it was not until the late 1960s that these techniques were widely and effectively employed in the treatment of this disorder. The reason can be found in the impact of the new psychoanalytical theory at the turn of this century. Soon after Janet gave his description of exposure therapy, Freud published his analysis of semantic conditioning in the formation of obsessions and compulsions in the patient known as the Rat Man (Freud, 1983), and interest turned toward the meaning of obsessions and compulsions and away from considering the compulsive behaviors as treatment targets themselves. A behavior therapist who has seen a large number of OCD patients would agree that the presentation of many of these cases appears to coincide with psychodynamic themes. However, although psychodynamic formulations have descriptive value, they have not yielded reliable techniques for modifying obsessions and compulsions. The need for direct behavioral treatment, even in cases that can also be explained in psychodynamic terms, finds support in an unexpected observation by Freud (1924) in discussing the psychoanalytic treatment of a related anxiety disorder: agoraphobia:

> Our technique grew up in the treatment of hysteria and is still directed principally to the cure of this affliction. But the phobias have made it necessary for us to go beyond our former limits. One can hardly master a phobia if one waits till the patient lets the analysis influence him to give it up . . . take the example of agoraphobia. It succeeds only when one can induce them through the influence of the analysis to behave like the first class, that is, to go out alone and to struggle with their anxiety while they are making the attempt. One first achieves therefore, a considerable moderation of the phobia and it is only when this has been attained by the physician's recommendation that the associations and memories come into the patient's mind, enabling the phobia to be solved.

Common Misconceptions About Behavior Therapy

In some cases, patients are not given behavior therapy due to long-standing misconceptions about this form of treatment. Corrections of the most common misconceptions are as follows: (1) behavior therapy will not lead to the formation of substitute symptoms; (2) interrupting compulsive rituals is not dangerous in any way to the patient; (3) the patient's thoughts and feelings are not ignored in behavior therapy; (4) behavior therapy no longer assumes that all maladaptive behavior is learned through simple conditioning processes; (5) the use of medication is not incompatible with behavior therapy; (6) behavior therapists recognize that their methods are not equally effective for all patients (Baer and Minichiello, 1986).

Outcome Studies

Controlled outcome studies of exposure and response prevention for OCD over the past 15 years, involving more than 200 patients in various countries, have found that 60–70 percent of patients with ritualistic behaviors were much improved after behavioral treatment. Approximately 20–30 percent of the patients were resistant to the treatment, and the dropout rate averaged 20 percent (Rachman and Hodgson, 1980; Marks, 1981; Rasmussen and Tsuang, 1984). Treatment was carried out over a relatively short period, averaging three to seven weeks, with a 10-session treatment program most common. At follow-up of two years or more, improvements in rituals were maintained in almost all of the patients (Marks, 1981). Patients with only obsessive thoughts, without ritualistic activity, were studied separately, with unpredictable results (Marks, 1981).

Foa et al. (1980) found that the exposure and response prevention components of behavior therapy may produce differential effects in the treatment of compulsive washers. Exposure therapy was found to help mainly in reducing the anxiety component, while response prevention was most effective in reducing the ritualistic washing. The combined treatment was more effective than either component in isolation. These authors also found that in treating checking rituals, a combination of imaginal exposure (i.e., having the patient vividly imagine the most feared consequences of not ritualizing) plus response prevention is superior to response prevention alone. This may be because the catastrophic consequences that many checkers fear will never occur in real life, so that habituation must be carried out in imagination (Foa et al., 1980).

The use of cognitive techniques in the treatment of obsessions and compulsions has been less predictable than the treatment consisting of exposure plus response prevention (Marks, 1981). Although the technique of thought stopping is widely used to treat obsessive thoughts, clear empirical support for its usefulness is lacking. Because OCD patients engage in obvious cognitive errors in inference and in assessing the probability of danger, the application of cognitive therapy techniques to change these cognitive processes directly would seem to be useful. However, the only controlled study in this area found that cognitive therapy did not add significantly to the therapeutic effects of exposure in vivo (Emmelkamp et al., 1980). This negative finding is consistent with the studies of other disorders treated with behavioral techniques: cognitive techniques do not add significantly to the results obtained with behavioral techniques aimed at the targeted behaviors (Latimer and Sweet, 1984).

Although obsessive and compulsive symptoms are usually greatly reduced with behavioral treatment, and interference with occupational and social functioning is reduced, the ritualistic behavior is rarely totally eliminated. As Marks (1981) has observed: "Although most patients who are cooperative (and those are the great majority) improve with exposure in vivo, few of them are totally cured. Patients are generally told that they need to acquire a coping set to deal with tendencies to ritualize that might recur after discharge. Occasionally brief booster treatment is needed, but this is minimal apart from explicit advice about regular homework, which may be needed for many months after discharge."

CONCLUSIONS

Initial Evaluation

The majority of OCD patients who present as treatment resistant have, in fact, not received appropriate treatment. The majority of clinician-referred OCD patients presenting to our clinic have never had trials of behavior therapy, and almost one-half have not undergone antidepressant trials.

In order to outline a treatment plan for an OCD patient, it is necessary to have a clear idea of exactly what the problem is, what exacerbates and what improves it, how it has evolved over the life of the patient, and what other symptoms and difficulties exist concomitantly. This optimally requires history taking that combines behavioral, psychodynamic, and family principles. To determine the appropriate treatment approach and understand the individual's potential for noncompliance, a thorough mental status examination is required. A depressed, manic, cognitively impaired, or psychotic patient requires a special treatment strategy. It is very unlikely that behavioral treatments will be effective until associated functional illnesses are well controlled. Also, alcoholic patients usually need treatment for alcoholism before they can comply with treatment aimed specifically at their obsessive-compulsive symptoms.

Medical Evaluation

It is extremely unusual for a medical or neurological illness to be associated with classical OCD. If *onset* of the illness occurs after age 50, the likelihood of associated disease probably increases. Possible neurological etiologies are reviewed elsewhere (Jenike, 1984b, 1986a).

Treatment

Patients with Only Obsessive Thoughts

In OCD patients who suffer from obsessive thoughts only and do not have rituals, a trial of antidepressant medication is a reasonable first choice. If available, start with clomipramine. Adequate trials may require as much as 250 mg/day for as long as ten to twelve weeks. Other antidepressants may also work, but they seem to be effective in a smaller percentage of patients. Newer agents, such as fluvoxamine and fluoxetine, may also turn out to be effective, and without some of clomipramine's troubling side effects. Fluoxetine is presently available in pharmacies in the United States. A number of studies are underway to evaluate the effectiveness of the newer agents.

Occasionally, obsessions improve within a few days. Anecdotal experience would indicate that MAOIs may be particularly rapid in terms of onset of effect.

Behavior therapy has little to offer the patient who does not have rituals. In those patients who are drug nonresponders, thought stopping, assertiveness training, systematic desensitization, imaginal flooding, and cognitive restructuring may be helpful in reducing symptoms.

Patients with Rituals

A few patients with compulsive rituals respond completely to either drugs or behavior therapy alone, but the majority require a combination of the two approaches for optimal clinical improvement. The techniques of exposure plus response prevention, as outlined earlier, are the mainstay of behavioral treatment. In patients with concomitant major depression, psychosis, or mania, it is unlikely that behavior therapy will be of help until these symptoms are well controlled pharmacologically. In such cases, initial treatment should be drug oriented, and behavior therapy should begin only after the affective or psychotic symptoms are optimally controlled.

In patients who perform rituals only at home, treatment must take place in the home. Family members need to function as surrogate therapists and supervise the exposure and response prevention. Many patients can be treated in an office setting, with homework given at the end of each session.

Patients with Personality Disorders

Assessment of personality disorders in OCD patients is important in predicting the outcome and determining the preferred treatment approach. As noted earlier, patients with severe personality disorders are largely refractory to the usual therapeutic strategies. These patients respond differently to previously validated behavioral techniques of exposure plus response prevention and are usually drug nonresponders. In particular, schizotypal personality disorder significantly impairs the treatment outcome and should be considered along with other predictors of poor outcome, such as severe depression, overvalued ideation, and noncompliance. This effect appears to be so strong that we recommend that outcome studies analyze data separately for patients who meet the criteria for this disorder and those who do not.

Until further data are available on the management of OCD patients with concomitant severe personality disorder, we manage them by focusing on reducing stress and conflict in their environments, which is best done with behavioral family or couples counseling. In addition, we attempt to arrange for day treatment, halfway house placement, or other alternative living arrangements away from the usually stressful environment where obsessive-compulsive symptoms often are exacerbated and reinforced. Once the stressful environment is eliminated, supportive therapy of these patients, with encouragement in exposure and response prevention and strong verbal reinforcement of the slightest gains, has been helpful to date in producing modest improvements in obsessions and compulsions. The long-term fate of these patients remains to be determined.

Medication Trials

Clomipramine is now available. Clinicians can also try fluoxetine, up to 80 mg/day. The optimal dosage for OCD is unknown, but a large multicenter trial is presently underway to determine this. Research centers may have access to agents with low toxicity that might be as effective as clomipramine and fluoxetine. If after trials of fluoxetine and clomipramine none of these drugs are available, any of the standard heterocyclic agents can be tried. Dosages should be in the antidepressant range, and blood levels may be helpful for imipramine, nortriptyline, and desipramine (Task Force, 1985). Response to any of the antidepressants may take ten to twelve weeks, and patients should be advised that medication trials cannot be evaluated if aborted for lack of efficacy until at least ten weeks have passed at therapeutic levels. Occasionally, patients respond earlier.

If two antidepressant trials fail or if the patient suffers concomitant panic attacks or severe anxiety, we generally proceed with a MAOI trial. Tranylcypromine, up to 60 mg daily, or phenelzine up to 90 mg daily, are the two drugs most commonly used.

Prior to changing the antidepressant medication, it is probably worthwhile to try to augment the response by adding lithium carbonate for a two- to four-week period. Based on case reports with clomipramine, this strategy occasionally yields positive results. Other agents that may augment the effect of fluoxetine include trazodone (100 mg at bedtime), clonazepine, buspirone, methylphenidate, and tryptophan. Definite recommendations concerning augmentation must await further data.

Anxiolytic agents are often used as adjuncts to other medications and may be helpful in facilitating behavior therapy in patients who are unable to tolerate the anxiety produced by exposure and response prevention techniques. It is unlikely that they will have a significant effect on OCD symptoms when used alone.

ECT or Psychosurgery

ECT is generally not helpful in OCD patients. However, in those patients who have a clear-cut depression that precedes the obsessive-compulsive symptoms, it may be worth trying.

From the collective data on psychosurgery, it appears that over one-half of the severe OCD patients improve. Postoperative personality changes are not evident with modern restricted operations, and surgical complications are few. A patient who has suffered for years with *extremely disabling* OCD that has responded poorly to more conventional therapies has a reasonable chance of achieving a favorable outcome, with relatively few risks. When more conservative treatments fail, psychosurgery is a viable option. Whether or not it will improve the clinical situation of the very severe OCD patient with a concomitant personality disorder is unknown.

REFERENCES

Altschuler M: Massive doses of trifluoperazine in the treatment of compulsive rituals. *Am J Psychiatry* 119:367, 1962.

Ananth J, Pecknold JC, van den Steen N, et al: Double-blind study of clomipramine and amitriptyline in obsessive neurosis. *Prog Neuropsychopharmacol* 5:257–262, 1981.

Ananth J, Solyom L, Bryntwick S, et al: Clomipramine therapy for obsessive compulsive neurosis. *Am J Psychiatry* 136:700–720, 1979.

Ananth J, Solyom L, Solyom C, et al: Doxepin in the treatment of obsessive compulsive neurosis. *Psychosomatics* 16:185–187, 1975.

Angst J, Theobald W: *Tofranil*. Berne, Switzerland, Verlag Stampfl, 1980, pp 11–32.

Annesley PT: Nardil response in a chronic obsessive compulsive. *Br J Psychiatry* 115:748, 1969.

APA Task Force Report No. 14 on Electroconvulsive Therapy. Washington, DC, American Psychiatric Association, 1978.

Baer L, Jenike MA, Ricciardi J, et al: Personality disorders in patients with obsessive-compulsive disorders. *Arch Gen Psychiatry* 47:826–832, 1990.

Baer L, Minichiello WE: Behavior therapy for obsessive-compulsive disorder, in Jenike MA, Baer L, Minichiello WE (eds): *Obsessive Compulsive Disorders: Theory and Management*. Littleton, MA, PSG Publishing Co, 1986, pp 45–76.

Baer L, Minichiello WE, Jenike MA: Behavioral treatment of obsessive-compulsive disorder with concomitant bipolar affective disorder. *Am J Psychiatry* 142:358–360, 1985.

Baer L, Minichiello WE, Jenike MA: Use of a portable-computer program in behavioral treatment of obsessive-compulsive disorder. *Am J Psychiatry* 144:1101, 1987.

Baer L, Minichiello WE, Jenike MA: Use of a portable-computer program to assist behavioral treatment in a case of obsessive-compulsive disorder. *J Behav Ther Psychiatry* 19:237–240, 1989.

Bailey HR, Dowling JL, Davies E: Cingulotomy and related procedures for severe depressive illness: studies in depression, IV, in Sweet WH, Obrador S, Martin-Rodriguez JG (eds): *Neurosurgical Treatment in Pain and Epilepsy*. Baltimore, University Park Press, 1975, pp 89–96.

Ballantine HT, Bouckoms AJ, Thomas EK, et al: Treatment of psychiatric illness by stereotactic cingulotomy. *Biol Psychiatry* 22:807–819, 1987.

Bauer G, Nowak H: Doxepine: Ein neues Antidepressivum Wirkungs-Verleich mit Amitriptyline. *Arzneimittelforsch* 19:1642–1646, 1969.

Bernstein IC, Callahan WA, Jaranson JM: Lobotomy in private practice. *Arch Gen Psychiatry* 32:1041–1047, 1975.

Bethume HC: A new compound in the treatment of severe anxiety states: Report on the use of diazepam. *N Engl J Med* 63:153–156, 1964.

Birley JLT: Modified frontal leucotomy: A review of 106 cases. *Br J Psychiatry* 110:211–221, 1964.

Black A: The natural history of obsessional neurosis, in Beech HR (ed): *Obsessional States*. London, Methuen & Co, 1974, pp 16–54.

Breitner C: Drug therapy in obsessional states and other psychiatric problems. *Dis Nerv Syst.* 21(suppl):31–35, 1960.

Bridges PK, Goktepe EO, Moratos J: A comparative review of patients with obsessional neurosis and depression treated by psychosurgery. *Br J Psychiatry* 123:663–674, 1974.

Brotman AW, Jenike MA: Monosymptomatic hypochondriasis treated with tricyclic antidepressants. *Am J Psychiatry* 141:1608–1609, 1984.

Capstick N: Clinical experience in the treatment of obsessional states. *J Int Med Res* 5(suppl 5):71–80, 1977.

Cole JO, Hartmann E, Brigham P: L-Tryptophan: Clinical studies. *McLean Hosp J* 5:37–71, 1980.

Coombe PD: Clomipramine and severe obsessive-compulsive neurosis. *Aust NZ J Psychiatry* 16:293–297, 1982.

De Montigny C, Grunberg F, Mayer A, et al: Lithium induces rapid relief of depression in tricyclic antidepressant drug non-responders. *Br J Psychiatry* 138:252–256, 1981.

De Veaugh-Geiss J, Landau P, Katz R: Treatment of obsessive compulsive disorder with clomipramine. *Psychiatr Ann* 19:97–101, 1989.

De Vorvrie GV: Anafranil (G34586) in obsessive neurosis. *Acta Neurol Belg* 68:787–792, 1968.

Diagnostic and Statistical Manual of Mental Disorders–Revised. Washington, DC, American Psychiatric Association, 1987.

Emmelkamp PMG, van der Helm M, van Zanten BL, et al: Treatment of obsessive-compulsive patients: The contribution of self-instructional training to the effectiveness of exposure. *Behav Res Ther* 18:61–66, 1980.

Epstein S, Jenike MA: Disabling urinary obsessions: An uncommon symptom of obsessive-compulsive disorder. Psychosomatics, in press.

Fernandez CE, Lopez-Ibor JJ: Monochlorimipramine in the treatment of psychiatric patients resistant to other therapies. *Actas Luso Esp Neurol Psiquiatr* 26:119–147, 1967.

Flament M, Rapoport JL: Childhood obsessive-compulsive disorder, in Insel TR (ed): *New Findings in Obsessive-Compulsive Disorder*. Washington, DC, American Psychiatric Association, 1984, pp 126–149.

Foa EB: Failure in treating obsessive-compulsives. *Behav Res Ther* 17:169–176, 1979.

Foa EB, Goldstein A: Continuous exposure and strict response prevention in the treatment of obsessive-compulsive neurosis. *Behav Ther* 17:169–176, 1978.

Foa EB, Steketee G, Milby JR: Differential effects of exposure and response prevention in obsessive-compulsive washers. *J Consult Clin Psychol* 48:71–79, 1980.

Fontaine R, Chouinard G: Antiobsessive effect of fluoxetine. *Am J Psychiatry* 142:989, 1985.

Forssman H, Walinder J: Lithium treatment of atypical indication. *Acta Psychiatr Scand* 207(Suppl):34–40, 1969.

Freud S: Turnings in the ways of psychoanalytic therapy, in *Collected Papers,* Vol. 2. London, Hogarth Press, 1924, pp 399–400. Originally published in 1919.

Freud S: *The Complete Psychological Works of Sigmund Freud,* Vols. 1–24, Strachey J (trans). London, Hogarth Press, 1983.

Geisler A, Schou M: Lithium ved tvangsneuroser. *Nord Psychiatr Tidsskr.* 23:493–495, 1970.

Geissman P, Kammerer T: L'imipramine dans la neurose obsessionelle: Etude de 39 cas. *Encephale* 53:369–382, 1964.

Goodman WK, Price LH, Rasmussen SA, et al: Efficacy of fluvoxamine in obsessive-compulsive disorder. *Arch Gen Psychiatry* 46:36–44, 1989.

Flament M, Rapoport JL: Childhood obsessive-compulsive disorder. In: *New Findings in Obsessive-Compulsive Disorder,* Insel TR (ed). Washington DC, American Psychiatric Press, 1984.

Foa EB, Goldstein A. (1978). Continuous exposure and strict response prevention in the treatment of obsessive-compulsive neurosis. Behav Ther. 17, 169–176.

Foa EB, Steketee G, Milby JR. (1980). Differential effects of exposure and response prevention in obsessive-compulsive washers. J Consult Clin Psychol. 48, 71–79.

Foa EB. (1979). Failure in treating obsessive-compulsives. Behav Res Ther. 17, 169–176.

Fontaine R, Chouinard G. (1985). Antiobsessive effect of fluoxetine. Am J Psychiatry. 142, 989.

Forssman H, Walinder J. (1969). Lithium treatment of atypical indication. Acta Psychiatr Scand Suppl. 207, 34–40.

Freud S. (1924). Turnings in the ways of psychoanalytic therapy. In: *Collected Papers.* London, Hogarth Press, vol. 2, pp 399–400. Originally published in 1919.

Freud S. (1983). *The Complete Psychological Works of Sigmund Freud,* vols. 1–24, Strachey J (trans). London, Hogarth Press, (1983).

Geisler A, Schou M. (1970). Lithium ved tvangsneuroser. Nord Psychiatr Tidsskr. 23, 493–495.

Geissman P, Kammerer T. (1964). L'imipramine dans la neurose obsessionelle: Etude de 39 cas. Encephale. 53, 369–382.

Goodman WK, Price LH, Rasmussen SA, et al. (1989). Efficacy of fluvoxamine in obsessive-compulsive disorder. Arch Gen Psychiatry. 46, 36–44.

Grabowski JR. (1968). Treatment of severe depression and obsessive depression with G3486. Folia Med. 57, 265–270.

Grimshaw L: The outcome of obsessional disorder: A follow-up study of 100 cases. *Br J Psychiatry* 111:1051–1056, 1965.

Gross M, Slater E, Roth M (eds): *Clinical Psychiatry.* Bailliere Tindall & Casel, 1969.

Gruber RP: ECT for obsessive-compulsive symptoms. *Dis Nerv Syst* 201–220, 1971.

Hussain MZ, Ahad A: Treatment of obsessive compulsive neurosis. *Can Med Assoc J* 103:648–650, 1970.

Insel TR, Murphy DL, Cohen RM, et al: Obsessive-compulsive disorder. A double-blind trial of clomipramine and clorgyline. *Arch Gen Psychiatry* 40:605–612, 1983.

Jain VK, Swinson RP, Thomas JE: Phenelzine in obsessional neurosis. *Br J Psychiatry* 117:237–238, 1970.

Janet P: *Les obsessions et la psychasthenie,* ed. 2. Paris, Bailliere, 1908.

Jenike MA: Rapid response of severe obsessive-compulsive disorder to tranylcypromine. *Am J Psychiatry* 138:1249–1250, 1981.

Jenike MA: Use of monoamine oxidase inhibitors in obsessive-compulsive disorder. *Br J Psychiatry* 140:159, 1982.

Jenike MA: A case report of successful treatment of dysmorphophobia with tranylcypromine. *Am J Psychiatry* 141:1463–1464, 1984a.

Jenike MA: Obsessive-compulsive disorder: A question of a neurologic lesion. *Compr Psychiatry* 25:298–304, 1984b.

Jenike MA: Illnesses related to obsessive-compulsive disorder, in Jenike MA, Baer L, Minichiello WE (eds): *Obsessive Compulsive Disorders: Theory and Management.* Littleton, MA, PSG Publishing Co, 1986a, pp 133–146.

Jenike MA: Predictors of treatment failure, in Jenike MA, Baer L, Minichiello WE (eds): *Obsessive Compulsive Disorders: Theory and Management.* Littleton, MA, PSG Publishing Co., 1986b, pp 125–132.

Jenike MA: Psychotherapy of the obsessional, in Jenike MA, Baer L, Minichiello WE (eds): *Obsessive Compulsive Disorders: Theory and Management,* Littleton MA, PSG Publishing Co, 1986c, pp 113–122.

Jenike MA: Somatic treatments, in Jenike MA, Baer L. Minichiello WE (eds): *Obsessive Compulsive Disorders: Theory and Management.* Littleton, MA, PSG Publishing Co., 1986d, pp 77–112.

Jenike MA: Theories of etiology, in Jenike MA, Baer L, Minichiello WE (eds): *Obsessive Compulsive Disorders: Theory and Management.* Littleton, MA, PSG Publishing Co, 1986e, pp 11–22.

Jenike MA: Coping with fear responses to AIDS. *Human Sexuality* 21:22–28, 1987.

Jenike MA, Armentano M, Baer L: Disabling obsessive thoughts responsive to antidepressants. *J Clin Psychopharmacol* 7:33–35, 1987a.

Jenike MA, Baer L: An open trial of buspirone in obsessive-compulsive disorder. *Am J Psychiatry* 145:1285–1286, 1988.

Jenike MA, Baer L, Minichiello WE, et al: Concomitant obsessive-compulsive disorder and schizotypal personality disorder: A poor prognostic indicator. *Arch Gen Psychiatry* 43:296, 1986a.

Jenike MA, Baer L, Minichiello WE, et al: Concomitant obsessive-compulsive disorder and schizotypal personality disorder. *Am J Psychiatry* 143:530–533, 1986b.

Jenike MA, Baer L, Minichiello WE: *Obsessive-Compulsive Disorders: Theory and Management.* Littleton, MA, PSG Publishing Co., 1986c.

Jenike MA, Baer L, Summergrad P, et al: Obsessive-compulsive disorder: A double-blind, placebo-controlled trial of clomipramine in 30 patients. *Am J Psychiatry* 146:1328–1330, 1989.

Jenike MA, Buttolph L, Baer L, et al: Fluoxetine in obsessive-compulsive disorder: A positive open trial. *Am J Psychiatry* 146:909–911, 1989.

Jenike MA, Pato C: Disabling fear of AIDS responsive to imipramine. *Psychosomatics* 27:143–144, 1986.

Jenike MA, Surman OS, Cassem NH, et al: Monoamine oxidase inhibitors in obsessive-compulsive disorder. *J Clin Psychiatry* 44:131–132, 1983.

Jenike MA, Vitigliano HL, Rabinovitz J, et al: Bowel obsessions: A variant of obsessive-compulsive disorder responsive to antidepressants. *Am J Psychiatry* 144:1347–1348, 1987b.

Jenike MA, Hyman SE, Baer I, et al: A controlled trial of fluoxamine for obsessive-compulsive disorder: Implications for a serotonergic theory. *Am J Psychiatry* 147:1209–1215, 1990.

Jiminez F: A clinical study of Anafranil in depressive, obsessional and schizophrenic patients. *Folia Neuropsiquat Sur Este Esp* 3:189, 1968.

Joel SW: Twenty month study of iproniazid therapy. *Dis Nerv Syst* 20:1–4, 1959.

Kahn RS, Westenberg HGM, Jolles J: Zimeledine treatment of obsessive-compulsive disorder. *Acta Psychiatr Scand* 69:259–261, 1984.

Kelly DHW, Walter C, Mitchell-Heggs N, et al: Modified leucotomy assessed clinically, physiologically and psychologically at six weeks and eighteen months. *Br J Psychiatry* 120:19–29, 1972.

Lader M, Wing L: Physiological measures in agitated and retarded depressed patients. *J Psychiatr Res* 7:89–100, 1969.

Latimer PR, Sweet AA: Cognitive versus behavioral procedures in cognitive-behavior therapy: A critical review of the evidence. *J Behav Ther Exp Psychiatry* 15:9–22, 1984.

Le Beau J: The cingular and precingular areas in psychosurgery (agitated behavior, obsessive compulsive states, epilepsy). *Acta Psychiatr Neurol Scand* 27:305–316, 1952.

Lopez-Ibor JJ: Intravenous infusions of monochlorimipramine. Technique and results, in *Proceedings of the Sixth International Congress of the CINP, Taragona, Spain, April 1968.* Exerpta Medica Foundation Int Congress Series No. 180. Amsterdam, 1969, pp 519–521.

Lydiard RB: Obsessive-compulsive disorder successfully treated with trazodone. *Psychosomatics* 27:858–859, 1986.

Marks IM: Review of behavioral psychotherapy, I: Obsessive-compulsive disorders. *Am J Psychiatry* 138:584–592, 1981.

Marks IM, Stern RS, Mawson D, et al: Clomipramine and exposure for obsessive compulsive rituals. *Br J Psychiatry* 136:1–25, 1980.

Marshall WK, Micev V: Clomipramine in the treatment of obsessional illness and phobic anxiety states. *J Int Med Res* 1:403–412, 1973.

Mellman LA, Gorman JM: Successful treatment of obsessive-compulsive disorder with ECT. *Am J Psychiatry* 141:596–597, 1984.

Minichiello WE, Baer L, Jenike MA: Schizotypal personality disorder: A poor prognostic indicator for behavior therapy in the treatment of obsessive-compulsive disorder. *J Anxiety Dis* 1:273–276, 1987.

Minichiello WE, Baer L, Jenike MA, et al: Age of onset of major subtypes of obsessive-compulsive disorder. *J Anx. Disorders,* 4:147–150, 1990.

Mitchell-Heggs N, Kelly D, Richardson A: Stereotactic limbic leucotomy: A follow-up at 16 months. *Br J Psychiatry* 128:226–240, 1976.

Montgomery SA: Clomipramine in obsessional neurosis: A placebo controlled trial. *Pharmacol Med* 1:189–192, 1980.

Myers JK, Weissman MM, Tischler GL, et al: Six month prevalence of psychiatric disorders in three commitments. *Arch Gen Psychiatry* 41:949–958, 1984.

O'Regan B: Treatment of obsessive compulsive neurosis with haloperidol. *Can Med Assoc J* 103:167–168, 1970a.

O'Regan B: Treatment of obsessive compulsive disorder, letter. *Can Med Assoc J* 103:648–650, 1970b.

Orvin GH: Treatment of the phobic obsessive compulsive patient with oxazepam, an improved benzodiazepine compound. *Psychosomatics* 8:278–280, 1967.

Perse TL, Griest JH, Jefferson JW, et al: Fluvoxamine treatment of obsessive-compulsive disorder. *Am J Psychiatry* 144:1543–1548, 1987.

Prasad AJ: Obsessive-compulsive disorder and trazodone. *Am J Psychiatry* 141:612–613, 1984.

Price LH, Goodman WK, Charney DS, et al: Treatment of severe obsessive-compulsive disorder with fluvoxamine. *Am J Psychiatry* 144:1059–1061, 1987.

Rachman SJ: *Fear and Courage*. San Francisco, WH Freeman, 1978.

Rachman SJ, Hodgson RJ: *Obsessions and Compulsions*. Englewood Cliffs, NJ, Prentice-Hall, 1980.

Rack PH: Clinical experience in the treatment of obsessed states. *J Int Med Res* 5(suppl 5):81–96, 1977.

Rasmussen SA: Lithium and tryptophan augmentation in clomipramine-resistant obsessive-compulsive disorder. *Am J Psychiatry* 141:1283–1285, 1984.

Rasmussen SA, Tsuang MT: The epidemiology of obsessive compulsive disorder. *J Clin Psychiatry* 45:450–457, 1984.

Rasmussen SA, Tsuang MT: Epidemiology and clinical features of obsessive-compulsive disorder, in Jenike MA, Baer L, Minichiello WE (eds): *Obsessive Compulsive Disorders: Theory and Management*. Littleton, MA, PSG Publishing Co, 1986b, pp 23–44.

Rimher Z, Szantok, Arato M, et al: Response of phobic disorders with obsessive symptoms to MAO inhibitors. *Am J Psychiatry* 139:1374, 1982.

Rivers-Buckeley N, Hollender MH: Successful treatment of obsessive-compulsive disorders with loxapine. *Am J Psychiatry* 139:1345–1346, 1982.

Robins LN, Helzer JE, Weissman MM, et al: Lifetime prevalence of specific psychiatric disorders in three sites. *Arch Gen Psychiatry* 41:958–967, 1984.

Smith B, Kilom LF, Cochrane N, et al: A prospective evaluation of open prefrontal leucotomy. *Med J Aust* 1:731–735, 1976.

Snyder S: Amitriptyline therapy of obsessive-compulsive neurosis. *J Clin Psychiatry* 41:286–289, 1980.

Solyom L, DiNicola VF, Phil M, et al: Is there an obsessive psychosis? Aetiological and prognostic factors of an atypical form of obsessive-compulsive neurosis. *Can J Psychiatry* 30:372–380, 1985.

Stern TA, Jenike MA: Treatment of obsessive-compulsive disorder with lithium carbonate. *Psychosomatics* 24:671–673, 1983.

Stroebel CF, Szarek BI, Glueck BC: Use of clomipramine in treatment of obsessive-compulsive symptomatology. *J Clin Psychopharmacol* 4:98–100, 1984.

Strom-Olsen R, Carlisle S: Bifrontal stereotactic tractotomy: A follow-up study of its effects in 210 patients. *Br J Psychiatry* 118:141–154, 1971.

Sturgis ET, Meyer V: Obsessive compulsive disorders, in Turner SM, Calhoun KC, Adams HE (eds). *Handbook of Clinical Behavior Therapy*. New York, John Wiley and Sons, 1980, pp 68–102.

Swinson RP: Response to tranylcypromine and thought stopping in obsessional disorder. *Br J Psychiatry* 144:425–427, 1984.

Sykes M, Tredgold R: Restricted orbital undercutting: A study of its effects on 350 patients over the ten years 1951–1960. *Br J Psychiatry* 110:609–640, 1964.

Tan E, Marks I, Marset P: Bimedial leucotomy in obsessive-compulsive neurosis: A controlled serial enquiry. *Br J Psychiatry* 118:155–164, 1971.

Task force on the use of laboratory tests in psychiatry: Tricyclic antidepressants—blood level measurements and clinical outcome. *Am J Psychiatry* 142:142–149, 1985.

Tesar GE, Jenike MA: Alprazolam as treatment for a case of obsessive-compulsive disorder. *Am J Psychiatry* 141:689–690, 1984.

Thoren P, Asberg M, Cronholm B, et al: Clomipramine treatment of obsessive compulsive disorder. I. A controlled clinical trial. *Arch Gen Psychiatry* 37:1281–1285, 1980a.

Thoren P, Asberg M, Cronholm B, et al: Clomipramine treatment of obsessive compulsive disorder. II. *Arch Gen Psychiatry* 37:1286–1294, 1980b.

Thyer BA, Parrish RT, Curtis GC, et al: Ages of onset of DSM-III anxiety disorders. *Compr Psychiatry* 26:113–122, 1985.

Tippin J, Henn FA: Modified leukotomy in the treatment of intractable obsessional neurosis. *Am J Psychiatry* 139:1601–1603, 1982.

Tollefson G: Alprazolam in the treatment of obsessive symptoms. *J Clin Psychopharmacol* 5:39–42, 1985.

Turner SM, Hersen M, Bellack AS, et al: Behavioral and pharmacological treatment of obsessive-compulsive disorders. *J Nerv Ment Dis* 168:651–657, 1980.

Van Putten T, Sander DG: Lithium in treatment failures. *J Nerv Ment Dis* 161:255–264, 1975.

Venkoba Rao A: A controlled trial with Valium in obsessive compulsive states. *J Indian Med Assoc* 42:564–567, 1964.

Walinder J, Skott A, Carlsson A, et al: Potentiation of the antidepressant action of clomipramine by tryptophan. *Arch Gen Psychiatry* 33:1384–1389, 1976.

Walter CJ, Mitchell-Heggs N, Sargant W: Modified narcosis, ECT, and antidepressant drugs: A review of technique and immediate outcome. *Br J Psychiatry* 120:651–652, 1972.

Waxman D: A clinical trial of clomipramine and diazepam in the treatment of phobic and obsessional illness. *J Int Med Res* 5(suppl 5):99–110, 1977.

Whitty CWM, Duffield JE: Anterior cingulectomy in the treatment of mental disease. *Lancet* 262:475–481, 1952.

Wyndowe J, Solyom L, Ananth J: Anafranil in obsessive compulsive neurosis. *Curr Ther Res* 18:611–617, 1975.

Yaryura-Tobias JA: Tryptophan may be adjuvant to obsessive-compulsive therapy. *Clin Psychiatr News* September 1981, 1981, p 16.

Yaryura-Tobias JA, Bhagavan HN: L-Tryptophan in obsessive-compulsive disorders. *Am J Psychiatry* 134:1298–1299, 1977.

Yaryura-Tobias JA, Neziroglu MS: The action of clorimipramine in obsessive compulsive neurosis: A pilot study. *Curr Ther Res* 17:1, 1975.

Yaryura-Tobias JA, Neziroglu MS, Bergman L: Clomipramine for obsessive compulsive neurosis: An organic approach. *Curr Ther Res* 20:541–548, 1976.

Yaryura-Tobias JA, Neziroglu MS, Bhagavan H: (1979). Obsessive-compulsive disorders: A serotonergic hypothesis, in Saletu B, Berner P, Hollister L (eds): *Neuropsychopharmacology: Proceedings of the 11th Congress of the CINP*. Oxford, Pergamon Press, 1979, pp 117–125.

8

Clinical Management of
Post-Traumatic Stress Disorder

JONATHAN DAVIDSON

Early reports of trauma-related psychiatric disturbances date back to the American Civil War (Mitchell et al., 1864), being referred to as "soldier's heart," "effort syndrome," and "neurasthenia." In World War I, interest again turned to the effect of war upon psychological functioning, and the term "shell shock" was coined (Mott, 1919). Shortly afterward (Drury, 1919; Wearn and Sturgis, 1919), biological challenge techniques were applied to the victims of combat, and evidence was adduced to suggest an enduring autonomic hyperarousal or physiological instability.

During the nineteenth century, the effect of railway injuries also received a great deal of attention, largely because of compensation issues. Many patients who suffered psychological symptoms following such injuries were diagnosed as suffering from "railway spine" (Trimble, 1981).

In World War II, Kardiner (1941) drew together the disparate reports describing the effects of trauma and recognized a common syndrome, which he termed "physioneurosis," as distinct from the more common term "psychoneurosis," and characterized this state as having the following five features: (1) a persistent startle response and irritability, (2) continued preoccupation with the trauma, (3) explosiveness and aggressive outbursts, (4) nightmares, and (5) constriction of interpersonal and social activities. These five features can be broadly subtyped into hyperarousal and numbing/withdrawal symptom clusters. Since the pioneering observations of Kardiner (1941), other investigators have described similar symptom clusters in civilian trauma victims, such as rape (Burgess and Holstrom, 1974), kidnapping (Terr, 1985), incest (Herman, 1983), and accidents (Wilkinson, 1983).

Diagnostically, the condition was first represented in DSM I as an acute stress reaction, subtyped into civilian and military forms. DSM I prohibited the existence of any preexisting psychiatric disorder and did not admit that stress disorder could become chronic. It stipulated that any traumatic reactions that became chronic did so because of more important preexisting conflicts. DSM II retained a place for traumatic reactions but discarded the military–civilian distinction, yet continued to view this as essentially an acute reaction. Moreover its importance was diminished in that it was equated with such reactions as the Ganser syndrome and a reaction to an unwanted pregnancy. DSM III approached the characterization and classification of traumatic stress reactions in more detail, probably being influenced by the recent experiences of veterans returning from Vietnam. In its characterization, post-traumatic stress disorder (PTSD) in DSM III closely resembled the description of Kardiner outlined above. In addition, a third cluster of symptoms was brought into the picture, namely, that of nonspecific hyperarousal. In the revision of DSM III, further modifications to the criteria have been made, but the essential tripartite division has persisted, along with the stipulation that the patient must have been exposed to a stress that is outside normal human experience and that would be expected to produce distress in almost anyone. A list of examples is given. Moreover, the acute form of PTSD, which was present in DSM III, has been dropped in the revision. A minimum duration of one month is required for the diagnosis.

MAGNITUDE OF THE PROBLEM

Recent epidemiological studies have indicated an approximately 1 percent lifetime prevalence of PTSD in a community (Helzer et al., 1987). Since this disorder is very often chronic, it may well be that 0.5 percent of the population has continued difficulty with symptoms relating to trauma. Furthermore, an additional 14–15 percent of the population have at some point experienced symptoms subsequent to the traumatic experience that fell short of meeting the full diagnostic criteria for PTSD.

Epidemiological reports from populations of Vietnam War veterans suggest that PTSD is more common, ranging from 2 to 15 percent. Another statistic that may give some idea of the magnitude of this problem is the fact that 8 percent of deaths in the United States result from unnatural causes. If one assumes an average of four surviving family members from such a bereavement, then 600,000 U.S. citizens might be expected to experience an unnatural bereavement each year (Rynearson, 1986). In regard to the number of returning Vietnam War veterans who may be in need of psychiatric help, estimates have ranged from 500,000 to 1.5 million (Walker and Cavenar, 1982). Incest, another precursor of traumatic stress reactions, has been reported in as many as 16 percent of the population (Herman et al., 1986).

Public awareness of PTSD has grown appreciably, as has the realization that it carries high morbidity and possibly even high mortality and that it may often become chronic. The study of treatment of PTSD remains at an early stage, and in some ways it lags behind our understanding of treatment for the other anxiety disorders. PTSD presents a unique set of challenges. The purpose of this chapter is to describe the recognition of PTSD, its differential diagnosis, and approaches to treatment.

DIAGNOSIS OF PTSD

As represented in DSM III-R, (American Psychiatric Association, 1987), the symptoms of PTSD are grouped into intrusive, avoidant, and hyperarousal constellations.

Intrusive events are as follows: (1) recurrent and intrusive, distressing recollections of the event; (2) recurrent distressing dreams of the event; (3) sudden acting or feeling as if the traumatic event were recurring; and (4) intense psychological distress at exposure to the events that symbolize or resemble an aspect of the trauma, including anniversaries thereof.

Avoidance features are as follows: (1) efforts to avoid thoughts or feelings associated with the trauma; (2) efforts to avoid activities or situations that arouse recollections of the trauma; (3) inability to recall an important aspect of the trauma (psychogenic amnesia); (4) markedly diminished interest in significant activities; (5) a feeling of detachment or estrangement from others; (6) a restricted range of affect; and (7) a sense of a foreshortened future.

Generalized hyperarousal may be indicated by any of the following: (1) difficulty falling or staying asleep; (2) irritability or outbursts of anger; (3) difficulty concentrating; (4) hypervigilance; (5) exaggerated startle response; and (6) physiological reactivity upon exposure to events that symbolize or resemble an aspect of the trauma. In order to qualify for the diagnosis of PTSD, the patient must have at least one intrusive symptom, three avoidant symptoms, and two hyperarousal features. Furthermore, the person must have experienced an event that is outside the range of usual human experience and that would be markedly distressing to almost anyone. Symptoms from the three groups must last for a minimum of one month, although it is not necessary that all three be present concurrently. Delayed PTSD is diagnosed if the symptoms first occurred at least six months after the trauma.

In a report by Horowitz et al. (1980), the frequency of key symptoms was assessed in patients who had presented at a stress disorders clinic following a recent acute trauma. Intrusive symptoms present in at least 75 percent of the subjects included the experience of waves of strong feeling about the trauma, sudden reminders through hearing or seeing things, thinking about it when the patient did not mean to do so, images repeatedly popping into the patient's mind, and any reminder bringing back emotions related to the trauma. Interestingly, nightmares were found in only 44 percent of the sample.

No single avoidant item was present in 75 percent of the sample, but the two most common ones were the realization that many unresolved feelings still existed but had been kept hidden and the avoidance of emotional upset when thinking about the trauma or being reminded of it.

In order to arrive at a diagnosis, it is first necessary to think about the possibility that a traumatic event might bear an important relationship to the patient's problem. While this may seem to be an obvious statement, it has been our experience that even trained psychiatrists frequently overlook trauma and PTSD in the history and therefore do not ask the patient about traumatic experiences. If a trauma has taken place, the physician would then need to review the three chief symptom groupings and rule out PTSD.

It is important to understand that patients with PTSD may not draw a connection between the trauma and their symptoms, but instead are likely to present with nonspecific complaints or problems related to a complicating diagnosis, such as depression or substance abuse. Patients often feel shameful or guilty about having been victimized and may repress unpleasant events. The painful feelings associated with the event may also be difficult for the patient to describe.

Although age appears not to govern the patient's symptoms in adulthood (Horowitz et al., 1980), children with PTSD may relive the trauma through play, may grow up with a sense of a foreshortened future such that they do not see themselves reaching adulthood, may develop a sense of foretelling the future (omen formation), and, while experiencing loss of interest and constricted affect, may have a hard time verbalizing it, so that it will be necessary to elicit observations from teachers or parents.

Sex does not seem to affect the symptom picture, although women may have higher scores than men on avoidant symptoms of PTSD (Horowitz et al., 1980).

In light of the above considerations, it is important to describe the ways in which PTSD can present and identify clues that might lead the physician to think more seriously about an underlying PTSD.

1. Somatic symptoms: Nonspecific somatic discomfort or preoccupations, headaches, and pain syndromes (Benedict and Kolb, 1986).
2. Sleep disturbance. A leading complaint about sleep disturbance should make one think of PTSD as a possible cause. This is even more likely if the patient describes graphic nightmares of real-life events and/or if he or she is unusually restless or agitated during the night or acts out dreams, such as by shouting or physically assaulting the sleeping partner. Any sleep disturbance that is severe enough to cause a sleeping partner to find it intolerable to share the bed should indicate PTSD as a possible diagnosis.
3. Irritability, explosiveness, unprovoked aggression.
4. Distancing and withdrawal from others. Increased isolation, sullenness, or frequent moodiness, especially if not in keeping with the patient's previous personality, should raise the suspicion of PTSD. These problems may well present in the form of marital discord or job instability.
5. Depression, suicidal ideas, or suicidal attempts.
6. High levels of anxious arousal or a physiological instability.
7. Antisocial behavior or violation of the law. When these changes occur for the first time in adulthood, it is less likely that they are related to an underlying character disorder and more likely that another Axis I illness, such as PTSD, might explain this behavior.

8. Substance or alcohol abuse. The physician can ask about the reason—
   for example, whether the patient finds it necessary to deaden painful
   memories and affect. This inquiry might lead to the question of PTSD.

PTSD is sometimes difficult to distinguish from antisocial personality
disorder. Bailey (1985) has described some of the distinguishing features
as follows. Favoring PTSD are the existence of a good premilitary adap-
tation, such as a good school record and involvement in extramural activities; joining the service for patriotic reasons or being drafted; a history
of combat and specific recollections of combat experiences; and onset of
symptoms in the postmilitary period. By contrast, with antisocial personality disorder, the following features are more likely: poor premorbid history, as reflected by truancy, antisocial behavior, and institutionalization;
being forced into the service or choosing it as an escape from an unpleasant set of circumstances; no history of combat or only vague recollections
thereof; and onset of symptoms throughout the premilitary and military
periods. In the current symptom picture of PTSD, one would look for
guilt, especially survivor guilt, preoccupation with changes within the
self, numbing of affect, and difficulty disclosing information about combat experiences, which may disappear only after trust has been established. On the other hand, with antisocial personality disorder, there is no
evidence of guilt, the patient's preoccupation concerns changes in the environment, strong feelings are disclosed largely for manipulative reasons,
and a high level of comfort exists in discussing the severity of the war
trauma.

Another important distinction to be made is that between true PTSD
and pseudo-PTSD. It is always important to ascertain that the patient was
indeed exposed to the trauma he claims to have endured, and the source
documentation should be reviewed. In the case of veterans, this can be
established by looking at the C file. Collateral history taking is also helpful here. Pseudo-PTSD itself falls into a number of different categories,
including lying, delusions, and combat-related symptoms insufficient for
a PTSD diagnosis (Hamilton, 1985).

Schizophrenia can sometimes be confused with PTSD. Walker and
Cavenar (1982) note the higher frequency of autistic features, delusions,
and formal thought disorder in the former category. In PTSD they em-
phasize the alternation between constricted and anxious affect; note that
psychotic symptoms are content specific, being related to the trauma; and
state that when the patient acts in a bizarre, "psychotic" fashion, it is
generally in response to a reminder of the inciting trauma.

The differential diagnosis may be aided by psychophysiological and
neuroendocrine measures. For example, Kosten et al. (1987) found that
veterans of PTSD could be distinguished from those with schizophrenia
and depression on the basis of elevated twenty-four-hour norepinephrine
and decreased urinary cortisol levels. Other investigators (Dobbs and Wilson, 1960; Blanchard et al., 1982; Pitman et al., 1987) have consistently
found that patients with PTSD can be distinguished from control veterans

or those with other psychiatric diagnoses by means of psychophysiological measures, such as heart rate, skin conductance, and electromyographic (EMG) activity, when measured in response to experimental situations in which the patient is reexposed to reminders or images of the original trauma. These conclusions have given rise to a psychophysiological hypothesis of PTSD (Kolb, 1987) that views the disorder as a conditioned pattern of abnormal arousal in response to any physically threatening event.

TREATMENT

General Principles

It is important that the physician win the patient's trust to help reduce the high levels of suspicion and paranoia often present. Many authorities (e.g., Wise, 1983; Ochberg, 1988) advocate focusing treatment on issues related to the trauma and the patient's attempts to deal with it. Probing for early conflict issues may be less productive. By focusing on the here and now, patients learn that they are seen as having inherently sound coping skills, and their strengths are reinforced.

Many different treatment approaches may be utilized. Perhaps the most frequent one is individual psychotherapy, but group therapy has been advocated as a particularly helpful modality (Walker and Cavenar, 1982) because the shared experiences may help victims to be better understood. Family therapy (Figley, 1988) and pharmacotherapy (Van der Kolk, 1987; Friedman, 1988) have also been used.

A common problem faced by victims is society's tendency to disbelieve their story and even to blame the victim. The great majority of Vietnam veterans, for example, returned to an environment that was nonempathic, rejecting, and disapproving.

Treatment may be slow to take effect, and the physician needs patience when undertaking the use of a particular technique in this illness.

Treatment of Acute Reactions

The principles for managing acute stress reactions can be summed up by the mnemonic BICEPS (Wise, 1983). That is to say, first, treatment should be *brief,* being completed within a few days. Second, it should be *immediate.* Fowlie and Aveline (1985) have shown that the victims of ejection from an airplane did better if they had access to immediate counseling. By delaying treatment, there is a greater chance that complications, secondary gain, and avoidance will set in. Third, it is best to provide a *central* location for treatment. For example, in the military setting, if the victims are given the same sort of treatment as other psychiatric patients, they are more likely to become permanently disabled. The fourth factor is *expectation,* i.e., the expectation that acute trauma victims will be able to return to good functioning and/or to the situation that originally provoked the traumatic reaction. A fifth consideration, is *proximity.* Treatment should be given as close to the combat zone as possible. The sixth element is *simplicity.* Treatment should be focused on the current problems, i.e., the trauma and the patient's response to it. These principles, while taken from observations in the military, may be applied to other acute traumatic stress reactions.

Drug therapy is helpful adjunctively at this stage. In particular, the use of sodium amytal may help uncover repressed and painful memories and experiences of the event.

Treatment of Chronic PTSD

Individual Therapy

A number of models have been proposed for understanding and approaching the treatment of PTSD. One of the better-known ones is that of Horowitz and co-workers (1980). The initial priority is to diminish the impact of external stress upon the patient and to equalize the patient's tendency to retreat, to withdraw, and to remain numb in the face of the intrusive distressing symptoms that are invariably present. All of this is undertaken to ultimately help the patient understand and integrate the meaning and experience of the trauma into his or her life, so that it is no longer experienced as though it were still happening.

Where the trauma has been milder and the patient has good coping skills, a stable support system, etc., such treatment may be successfully accomplished in a limited time. However, more long-lasting trauma, severe symptoms, and disruption of the patient's life may be more suitably managed with a longer term of therapy. Ochberg (1988) distinguishes between treatment directed at pretrauma pathology and treatment directed around the trauma, the latter of which he refers to as "posttraumatic therapy." Five paradigms are identified to explain the symptom picture components. The first of these, *bereavement,* is obviously relevant if someone has been killed or lost as a result of the trauma; successful management will facilitate the formation of new attachments. The second factor is *victimization.* A victimized patient has to deal with low self-esteem and feelings of humiliation. Those feelings are often fueled by misunderstanding or disbelief on the part of others. Ochberg has suggested that this paradigm is not sufficiently well recognized or represented in our language. *Autonomic arousal* is present as part of PTSD as long as the illness remains active and as long as the patient experiences internal or external remainders of the trauma. A number of distressing physical symptoms arise from autonomic instability. *Physical injury* is often present in patients with PTSD. The fifth concept, *negative intimacy,* is especially applicable to patients whose trauma results from having been violated in the course of a close relationship. Negative intimacy is an important concept in understanding the victims of rape, assault, brutality, and kidnapping. Also relevant here is the war veteran with PTSD who has been involved in the perpetration of brutalizing acts in wartime.

Group Treatment

Walker and Cavenar (1982) have described the unique advantages of group therapy in PTSD. It is necessary for the therapist to tolerate highly charged and intense affect and to remain emotionally neutral when hearing about horrifying or disgusting experiences; it is important not to take sides. Participating in the group can help victims find others with the same depth of understanding, perhaps to initiate new attachments and to find meaning for the traumatic experience.

Another group therapy approach, as described by Flannery (1987), consists of small groups that meet for eight sessions, again emphasizing here-and-now issues. This treatment technique can best be described as a stress management/behavior modification intervention. After an initial didactic account of stress and stress reactions, work proceeds on the following goals: dietary modification (reduced intake of refined sugar, caffeine, and nicotine), hard exercise every day (e.g., brisk walks for twenty to thirty minutes), the development of relaxation techniques, and the development of stress inoculation skills. With the last intervention, patients anticipate stressful situations ahead of time and plan how to approach them, perhaps calling upon some of the other skills they have been taught. Flannery points out that this treatment approach is particularly helpful in dealing with the negative/avoidant symptoms of PTSD—the passivity, demoralization, and learned helplessness. The point is made that patients who can take more control over their own lives and environments are in a better position to maximize treatment effects. The learned helplessness model (Van der Kolk, 1987) of PTSD posits that, among other things, the victim has reached a position from which he or she feels unable to influence the environment or to shape his or her own life.

Individual therapy can be helpful in conjunction with group treatment, and it is often necessary for the patient to relive and face the traumatic experience within therapy. Details of traumatic events are frequently unpleasant and may evoke resistance on the part of the therapist as well as the patient. Individual therapy also provides the opportunity to explore the meaning of the trauma for the patient.

Flooding and desensitization approaches have been used in the behavioral management of PTSD.

It is important to judge whether, for a certain patient, it is best to uncover the trauma and help the patient to reintegrate the experience, albeit with increased levels of distress at various times of treatment, or whether it is preferable to seal over this aspect and enable the patient to direct his or her energy to current life issues and coping. Most likely there are some individuals for whom such uncovering is counterproductive.

Family Therapy

Figley (1988) has described the use of family treatment for patients with PTSD. Ways in which family members might facilitate the recovery process are as follows. (1) They may identify the traumatic stress by virtue of alterations in victim's behavior. Family members are in a good position to detect uncharacteristic actions. (2) They can encourage confrontation of the trauma. This can be done in a number of ways. (3) Understanding family members can urge recapitulation of the catastrophe by assisting the victim to recall different aspects of the trauma in such a way as to help answer four key questions: What happened? Why did it happen? Why did the person act in a particular way? and What would the person do in the future if a similar event happened again? (4) They can facilitate resolution of conflict.

Pharmacotherapy

Barbiturates and medicine were used in World War II for the abreactive treatment of acute PTSD (Sargant and Slater, 1972). These same authors also made the interesting, now entirely neglected, observation that patients with chronic PTSD may respond to 30 percent CO_2 inhalations. Somatic treatment of PTSD remained unexplored until a report of the successful use of phenelzine in five patients (Hogben and Cornfield, 1981).

Drugs can be useful in managing PTSD in the following ways: (1) to decrease the general hyperarousal and vigilance that characterize the syndrome; (2) to promote improved sleep and to control nightmares; (3) to provide greater distance between the patient and the emotional impact of the trauma; (4) to improve the patient's mood and relieve depression, suicidality, and anhedonia; (5) to enhance control over impulses of aggression and violence; and (6) to control psychotic manifestations when these are present. Since the objectives can be diverse, it is not surprising that many different drugs may be useful, and at times patients might need multiple-drug therapy. Each of the chief drug groups will be reviewed.

Tricyclics

There are five known reports of trycyclic therapy in veterans of Vietnam or World War II, one report in civilian accident victims, and one report in Israeli veterans (White, 1983; Burstein, 1984; Falcone et al., 1985; Lipper et al., 1986; Bleich et al., 1987; Frank et al., 1988; Wolf et al., 1988). Most of these studies were uncontrolled and used rudimentary measures for assessing the outcome. The report of Burstein (1984) included the Impact of Events Scale (IOES) and found that imipramine was effective for intrusive but not avoidant symptoms of PTSD and accident victims. Others (Embry and Callahan, 1988; Davidson et al., unpublished data) have noted that decreased libido is a TCA (tricyclic antidepressant) responsive symptom in PTSD.

Lipper et al. (1986) found carbamazepine useful in treating Vietnam veterans, particularly their symptoms of hostility, flashbacks, and nightmares. Carbamazepine is of particular interest in PTSD, since it may be effective in decreasing the intrusive symptoms by virtue of its antikindling property, and calls to mind Antelman's model (Antelman, 1988) of PTSD as arising from stress-induced sensitization. Van der Kolk (1987) suggested that repeated traumatization can give rise to lasting neurobiological and behavioral changes through kindling. Wolf et al. (1988) reported confirmatory findings in 18 patients with PTSD who received carbamazepine.

The study by Falcone and colleagues (1985) was uncontrolled, but the authors found that the presence of concomitant substance or alcohol abuse reduced the benefit of therapeutic drugs.

In a preliminary double-blind study, Frank and associates (1988) indicated that imipramine was associated with a higher overall improvement rate than placebo in a population of Vietnam veterans attending an outreach center. The strengths of this study are the use of standardized rating scales, and the careful monitoring of plasma levels.

The Israeli study (Bleich et al., 1987) described the clinical response anecdotally. Of interest is the high success rate (85 percent) with amitriptyline when the treatment was continued for six months. The authors believe that drug effects are more pronounced when drugs are administered in conjunction with psychotherapy.

Monoamine Oxidase Inhibitors

Phenelzine is the most intensively studied drug for the treatment of PTSD. Following the report of Hogben and Cornfield (1981), Davidson et al. (1987) demonstrated the benefit of phenelzine in 7 of 11 patients with PTSD. Although the doses were relatively low (45–60 mg), patient tolerance of phenelzine was not very good; dizziness, disruption of the sleep-wake cycle, and sexual impairment were reported. On the other hand, intrusive recollections, constricted affect, detachment/estrangement, and impaired memory or concentration improved with the drug. The maximum response was present at the end of two weeks, a pattern often seen when placebo is administered.

Additional studies with phenelzine include a controlled crossover trial matching the drug with placebo in 10 Israeli veterans (Shestatsky et al., 1988). Their results revealed no drug effect, but there was evidence of a time effect. Lerer et al. (1987) evaluated phenelzine in 22 Israeli combat veterans in an open trial and also found only weak drug effects on several standardized rating scales.

In the double-blind evaluation of phenelzine, imipramine, and placebo (Frank et al., 1988), preliminary analysis revealed that phenelzine was more effective than placebo and as effective as imipramine, with a suggestion of greater benefit with intrusive symptoms.

Other Drugs

Kolb et al. (1984) report improvement with clonidine and propranolol. Both treatments were associated with improvements in intrusive reexperiencing, nightmares, explosiveness, and autonomic hyperarousal. Moreover, the patients developed an enhanced sense of well-being and confidence and greater control over their physiology. Clonidine was administered in a dose of 0.2 to 0.4 mg/day, and propranolol was administered in doses of up to 180 mg/day. Van der Kolk (1983; 1987) has also noted effects of propranolol at high doses, but often such doses produce symptoms of organic brain syndrome.

An unpublished study by Lerer et al. indicates no superiority for alprazolam over placebo on PTSD symptoms in a double-blind crossover trial, although the drug did reduce general symptoms of anxiety, as measured on the Hamilton Anxiety Scale.

The place of lithium remains to be more clearly defined. Van der Kolk (1983) reports success in 14 patients; this author has also noted improvement with the drug, especially on symptoms of explosiveness, irritability, mood swings, and impaired sleep. Lithium is helpful in PTSD regardless of whether the patient has a personal or family history of bipolar disorder. However, when there is such a history, the place of the drug is more clearly defined.

Neuroleptics have not been well studied in PTSD, and their potential to develop tardive dyskinesia is an obvious limitation when drugs are given chronically. However, for short-term use in the management of psychotic features, they may well have a place.

One important point to remember in the pharmacotherapy of PTSD is that the response is usually relatively slow. In contrast to conditions like panic disorder and major depression, the response to drug therapy in PTSD is slower. In a placebo-controlled trial completed by the author (Davidson et al., unpublished data), amitriptyline did not become superior to placebo until week 80. The six-month treatment period of Bleich et al. (1987) has already been mentioned, as has the ten-week time effect noted in the study of phenelzine by Shestatsky et al. (1988). In this regard, the treatment response is more like that of obsessive/compulsive disorder, namely, slow and circumscribed. Since most clinical trials have been undertaken in patients with chronic symptoms, it would be instructive to learn whether residual symptoms are fewer in patients who have a short duration of illness and who are given vigorous pharmacotherapy. We do have evidence that both intrusive and avoidance symptoms of PTSD, as measured by the IOES, respond to drug therapy.

In many cases PTSD is masked by some other pathology, such as depression, suicidal behavior, alcohol or substance abuse, or antisocial behavior. These problems must be addressed before attempts are made to treat PTSD. When depression is very severe, the author has seen a good response to electroconvulsive therapy. However, the underlying PTSD may well persist, in which case appropriate treatment is required.

Other Treatments

Support groups represent one of the most helpful treatment modalities. Former prisoners of war or combat veterans often do well in groups with others who have undergone the same traumatic experiences. The same can be said for abused women or for victims of incest or rape. However, while it is beneficial for many patients, not everyone feels comfortable in the group format, and the patient should be given a choice in this matter.

Educational strategies are also helpful. Public awareness of PTSD is still inadequate; a description of its features and simple explanations using either biological or psychological models also have a place. Supportive treatment might be necessary for the spouse or other significant family members. The pathogenic effect upon a child whose parent has PTSD should be remembered as well (Rosenheck, 1985). We have found an unusually high incidence of psychopathology, including attention deficit, in the children of Vietnam veterans with PTSD (Davidson et al., unpublished data).

Conclusions

In PTSD it is important to initiate treatment as early as possible. When the stressful event is not too severe or chronic, a time-limited treatment of three to four months can accomplish much. In more chronic stresses, more overwhelming trauma, and if the patient's coping skills were deficient prior to the trauma, treatment is more likely to be time unlimited. If personality disorder is present, then as with most other Axis I disorders (e.g., depression), the treatment response is less favorable. The relative merits of different treatment approaches, as well as the ways in which they may interact in complementary fashion, need further study. The phasic course of PTSD should also be recalled, since patients may remain well for many years but experience a flareup of symptoms at the time of a life change (e.g., retirement or bereavement), which revives the affects associated with the original trauma.

REFERENCES

Antelman SM: Time-dependent sensitization as the cornerstone for a new approach to pharmacotherapy: Drugs as foreign/stressful stimuli. *Drug Dev Res* 14:1–30, 1988.
Bailey JE: Differential diagnosis of post traumatic stress disorder and antisocial personality disorders. *Hosp Community Psychiatry* 36:881–883, 1985.
Benedict RA, Kolb LC: Preliminary findings on chronic pain and post traumatic stress disorder. *Am J Psychiatry* 143:908–910, 1986.
Blanchard EB, Kolb LC, Pallmeyer TP, et al: A psychophysiological study of

post traumatic stress disorder in Vietnam veterans. *Psychiatr Q* 54:220–229, 1982.

Bleich A, Siegel B, Garb B, et al: Post traumatic stress disorder following combat exposure: Clinical features and psychopharmacological treatment. *Br J Psychiatry* 149:365–369, 1987.

Burgess AW, Holstrom L: Rape trauma syndrome. *Am J Psychiatry* 131:981–986, 1974.

Burstein A: Treatment of post-traumatic stress disorder with imipramine. *Psychosomatics* 25:681–686, 1984.

Davidson JRT, Walker JI, Kilts CD: A pilot study of phenelzine in the treatment of post traumatic stress disorder. *Br J Psychiatry* 150:250–255, 1987.

Diagnostic and Statistical Manual of Mental Disorders, ed 3 rev. Washington, DC, American Psychiatric Association, 1987.

Dobbs D, Wilson WP: Observations on the persistence of war neurosis. *Dis Nerv Syst* 21:40–46, 1960.

Drury AN: The percentage of carbon dioxide in the alveolar air, and the tolerance to accumulating carbon dioxide, in cases of so-called "irritable heart" of soldiers. *Heart* 17:165–173, 1919.

Embry CK, Callahan B: Effective pharmacotherapy for post traumatic stress disorder. *VA Practitioner* 5:57–66, 1988.

Falcone S, Ryan C, Chamberlain K, et al: Tricyclics: Possible treatment of post traumatic stress disorder. *J Clin Psychiatry* 46:385–389, 1985.

Figley CR: Post-traumatic family therapy, in Ochberg F (ed): *Post Traumatic Therapy and Victims of Violence.* New York, Brunner-Mazel, 1988, pp 102–125.

Flannery RB: From victim to survivor: A stress management approach in the treatment of learned helplessness, in Van der Kolk BA (ed): *Psychological Trauma.* Washington, DC, American Psychiatric Association Press, 1987, pp 217–232.

Fowlie DG, Aveline MO: The emotional consequences of ejection, rescue and rehabilitation in Royal Air Force air crew. *Br J Psychiatry* 146:609–613, 1985.

Frank JB, Kosten TR, Giller EL, et al: A randomized trial of phenelzine and imipramine for post traumatic stress disorder. *Am J Psychiatry* 145:1289–1291, 1988.

Friedman MJ: Toward rational pharmacotherapy for post traumatic stress disorder: An interim report. *Am J Psychiatry* 145:281–285, 1988.

Hamilton J de V: Pseudo-post traumatic stress disorder. *Milit Med* 150:353–356, 1985.

Hearst N, Newman TB, Hulley SB: Delayed effect of the military draft on mortality: A randomized natural experiment. *N Engl J Med* 314:620–624, 1986.

Helzer JE, Robins LN, McEvoy L: Post-traumatic stress disorder in the general population: Findings from the Epidemiological Catchment Area Survey. *N Engl J Med* 317:1630–1634, 1987.

Herman J: (1986). Histories of violence in an outpatient clinic. *Am J Psychiatry* 57:137–141, 1986.

Herman J, Russell D, Trocki K: Long term effects of incestuous abuse in childhood. *Am J Psychiatry* 143:1293–1296, 1986.

Hogben GL, Cornfield RB: Treatment of traumatic war neurosis with phenelzine. *Arch Gen Psychiatry* 38:440–445, 1981.

Horowitz MJ, Wilner N, Kaltreider N, et al: Signs and symptoms of post traumatic stress disorder. *Arch Gen Psychiatry* 37:85–92, 1980.

Kardiner A: *The Traumatic Neuroses of War.* New York, Hoeber, 1941.

Kolb LC: Neurophysiological hypotheses explaining post traumatic stress disorders. *Am J Psychiatry* 144:989–995, 1987.

Kolb LC, Burris BC, Griffiths S: Propranolol and clonidine in the treatment of post traumatic stress disorders of war, in Van der Kolk BA (ed): *Post Traumatic Stress Disorders: Psychological and Biological Sequelae.* Washington, DC, American Psychiatric Association Press, 1984, pp 29–42.

Kosten TR, Mason JW, Giller EL, et al: Sustained urinary norepinephrine and epinephrine elevations in post traumatic stress disorder. *Psychoneuroendocrinology* 12:13–20, 1987.

Lerer B, Bleich A, Kotler M, et al: Post traumatic stress disorders in Israeli combat veterans. *Arch Gen Psychiatry* 44:976–981, 1987.

Lipper SL, Davidson JRT, Grady TA, et al: Preliminary study of carbamazepine in post traumatic stress disorder. *Psychosomatics* 27:849–854, 1986.

Mitchell SW, Morehouse TS, Keen WS: *Gunshot Wounds and Other Injuries of Nerves.* Philadelphia, JB Lippincott Co, 1864.

Mott FW: *War Neuroses and Shell Shock.* London, Oxford Medical Publications, 1919.

Ochberg FM: Post traumatic therapy and victims of violence, in Ochberg F (ed): *Post Traumatic Therapy and Victims of Violence.* New York, Brunner-Mazel, 1988, pp 214–223.

Pitman RK, Orr SP, Foegue SP, et al: Psychophysiologic assessment of post traumatic stress disorder imagery in Vietnam combat veterans. *Arch Gen Psychiatry* 44:970–975, 1987.

Rosenheck R: Impact of post-traumatic stress disorder of World War II in the next generation. *J Nerv Ment Sci* 174:319–327, 1986.

Rynearson EK: (1986). Psychological effects of unnatural dying and bereavement. *Psychiatr Ann* 16:272–276, 1986.

Sargant WW, Slater E: *An Introduction to Physical Methods of Treatment in Psychiatry.* New York, Science Home, 1972, pp 149–157.

Shestatsky M, Greenberg D, Lerer B: A controlled trial of phenelzine in post traumatic stress disorder. *Psychiatry Res* 24:149–155, 1988.

Terr L: Chowchilla revisited: The effects of psychic trauma four years after a school bus kidnapping. *Am J Psychiatry* 140:1543–1550, 1983.

Trimble MR: The beginning-railway spine, in Trimble MR (ed): *Post Traumatic Neurosis.* New York, John Wiley and Sons, 1981, pp 40–59.

Van der Kolk BA: Psychopharmacological issues in post traumatic stress disorders. *Hosp Community Psychiatry* 34:683–684, 1983.

Van der Kolk BA: The drug treatment of post-traumatic stress disorder. *J Affective Disord* 13(2):203–213, 1987.

Walker JI, Cavenar JO: Forgotten warriors: Continuing problems of Vietnam veterans, in Cavenar JO, Brodie HKH (eds): *Critical Problems in Psychiatry.* Philadelphia, JB Lippincott Co., 1982, pp 161–175.

Wearn JT, Sturgis CC: Studies on epinephrine: Effects of the injection of epinephrine in soldiers with "irritable heart." *Arch Intern Med* 24:247–259, 1919.

White NS: Post traumatic stress disorder. *Hosp Community Psychiatry* 34:1061, 1983.

Wilkinson CB: Aftermath of a disaster, collapse of Hyatt Regency Hotel sky-walks. *Am J Psychiatry* 140:1134–1139, 1983.

Wise MG: Post traumatic stress disorder: The human reaction to catastrophe. *Drug Ther* 3:97–105, 1983.

Wolf ME, Alavi A, Mosnaim ME: Post traumatic stress disorder in Vietnam veterans. Clinical and EEG findings: Possible therapeutic effects of carbamazepine. *Biol Psychiatry* 23:642–644, 1988.

9

Treatments of Choice
for Anxiety Disorders

RUSSELL NOYES, JR.

Remarkable progress has been made in the treatment of anxiety disorders over the past decade. Looking at Figures 9–1 and 9–2, which list the most effective treatments for individual disorders, one sees pharmacological and behavioral strategies that are quite varied. Most are backed by carefully controlled studies establishing their usefulness and their superiority to competing treatments, although much work needs to be done. Nonetheless, a recent survey of practicing psychiatrists revealed that there was little agreement about how patients with anxiety disorders should be treated and even less agreement with experts in the field (Andrews et al., 1987). This disagreement should no longer exist because there is sufficient evidence for consensus. Taking this evidence into account, this chapter will outline the treatment approach to patients with anxiety disorders, as defined in DSM III-R (American Psychiatric Association, 1987). It will identify the treatments of choice and indicate how these should be administered for each disorder. It will also describe alternative treatments and indicate when these might be selected. Before discussing specific therapies, however, it will address several issues that influence our approach to treatment.

ISSUES IN TREATMENT

Diagnosis is the key to appropriate treatment, as indicated in Figures 9–1 and 9–2. These figures reveal a certain amount of treatment specificity. If their choices were limited to a single therapy, present-day therapists might select imipramine or exposure in vivo. Yet these treatments, either singly or combined, are useful for some anxiety disorders but not others. There is a good deal of uncertainty about the classification of these disorders, which naturally complicates the choice of treatment (Noyes, 1988c). For example, debate continues over the relationship between anxiety and depression; some claim that they are independent, while others

140

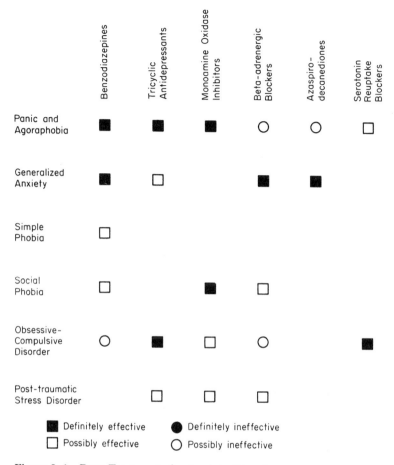

Figure 9–1   Drug Treatments for Anxiety Disorders.

believe that they share a common vulnerability (Stavrakaki and Vargo, 1986). The co-occurrence of anxiety and alcohol-related disorders has prompted similar questions about the interaction between these illnesses (Ross et al., 1988). Also, because of the overlap between anxiety disorders, the boundaries between them remain poorly defined. For example, the relationships between panic disorder and agoraphobia, as well as between panic and generalized anxiety disorder, have yet to be clarified (Noyes, 1986).

Knowledge about the course and outcome of anxiety disorders is critical to our assessment of the benefits and risks of various treatments. Unfortunately, information of this kind, especially for the newly defined anxiety disorders, is limited. Available evidence indicates that, for those who become psychiatric patients, the illnesses are chronic (Noyes, 1988a). This means that most treatments, while beneficial, do not cure the patients, who thus remain symptomatic. Further, it means that when the

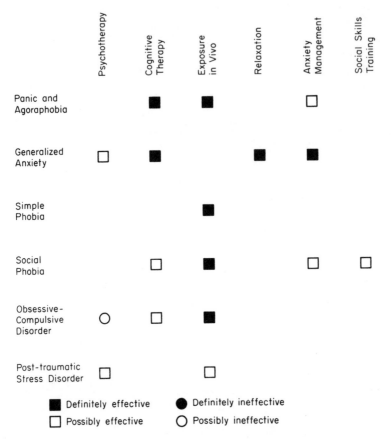

Figure 9–2 Psychological Therapies for Anxiety Disorders.

treatments are discontinued, symptoms may return to pretreatment levels. Under these circumstances, patients who have been placed on drugs tend to remain on them (Noyes et al., 1989a). It therefore becomes important to know what long-term benefits and risks these treatments have.

Proponents of behavioral therapies claim that their approach is superior in the long run. They point out that patients who have benefited from exposure maintain improvement over long periods of time, whereas patients who have benefited from drugs relapse when they are discontinued. A series of studies, following up agoraphobics treated with exposure in vivo, have shown gains maintained for five or more years (Lelliott et al., 1987). In addition, patients treated in this manner are not exposed to the long-term risks of drug treatment, including dependence on benzodiazepines and adverse effects such as weight gain, increased blood pressure, and even seizures with the tricyclic antidepressants (Noyes et al., 1988c; Noyes et al., 1989a). However, because there have been no studies directly comparing the long-term effects of drug and behavior therapies, we cannot be sure about their relative risks and benefits.

The relative efficacy of drug and behavioral treatments is a matter of great importance. Both have proven highly efficacious in controlled studies. However, there are almost no studies comparing these types of intervention with one another, so the question of which is more effective remains unanswered. Because psychologists usually employ behavioral therapies and psychiatrists administer drugs, this issue easily becomes the focus of a territorial dispute. Certainly, we do not wish to give drugs to patients who may be treated just as well without them. On the other hand, we do not wish to deny effective drug treatment to persons because of an unwarranted bias against such interventions. There is now evidence, at least in panic disorder and agoraphobia, of a positive interaction between drug and behavior therapies (Mavissakalian, 1988). For this reason, these therapies should usually be combined. At the least, both should be available to patients who might benefit from them.

REASONS FOR TREATMENT FAILURE

Before considering the treatments of choice, some reasons for treatment failure should be noted. The first of these is incorrect diagnosis. Anxiety symptoms are frequently present in many psychiatric illnesses. However, when these symptoms are emphasized or offered as presenting complaints, other diagnoses may be missed. Twenty percent of patients with major depression experience panic attacks, a symptom cluster that may lead the diagnostician astray (Coryell et al., 1988). Also, within the anxiety disorders there is overlap of symptoms, and separation of disorders is often based on rather fine distinctions. For example, the difference between social phobia and agoraphobia lies not only in the setting in which anxiety occurs but also in what the phobic person believes might go wrong. Consequently, careful history taking and diagnostic assessment are critical to treatment success.

Another reason for treatment failure is inadequate treatment. Of course, a treatment may be inadequate because it is the wrong approach for a particular disorder. There is no evidence that intensive psychotherapy works for obsessive-compulsive disorder, for example (Jenike, 1986). A treatment may also be inadequate if it is administered in a half-hearted manner. Unless a patient with panic disorder with agoraphobia has received at least 200 mg of imipramine for six weeks, he or she cannot be said to have had an adequate trial of this drug (Zitrin et al., 1983). Finally, treatment may be inadequate when it is not combined with other treatments that are known to be effective. As stated earlier, drug and behavior approaches should usually be employed together, and nonspecific factors (e.g., education, support) should be emphasized because many patients are strongly influenced by them.

Another reason for treatment failure has to do with associated features or problems. In general, patients who meet criteria for more than one disorder tend to have more severe illnesses that respond less well to treatment. But certain co-morbidities seem especially important. Patients who suffer from alcohol dependence in addition to an anxiety disorder are unlikely to respond to treatment for the latter until they become abstinent. Obsessive-compulsive disorder patients who also have depression are not likely to respond well to behavior therapy (Baer and Minichiello, 1986). Also, panic patients with obsessions and compulsions respond less well to treatment than those without these symptoms (Mellman and Uhde, 1987). In addition, the presence of a personality disorder may make treatment more difficult and less effective. Stressful life circumstances (e.g., marital conflict, job dissatisfaction), lack of social support, and secondary gains of illness may contribute to treatment failure.

TREATMENTS OF CHOICE

Panic Disorder

The current treatment of choice for panic disorder is imipramine, as shown in Table 9–1. Although phenelzine and alprazolam appear equally effective, imipramine appears to be safer and free of dependence potential (Noyes et al., 1986). A few patients respond to less than 100 mg daily, but others require 200 mg or more to bring them into the therapeutic range (Mavissakalian and Pevel, 1989). Of those who tolerate the drug, nearly 80 percent report at least moderate improvement and most become free

Table 9–1   Drug and Psychological Therapies of Choice for Anxiety Disorders

Disorder	Drug Therapies	Psychological Therapies
Panic disorder	Imipramine Phenelzine Alprazolam	Cognitive therapy Anxiety management
Agoraphobia	Imipramine	Exposure in vivo Cognitive therapy
Generalized anxiety disorder	Diazepam Buspirone	Relaxation, etc. Cognitive therapy Anxiety management
Simple phobia		Exposure in vivo
Social phobia	Phenelzine Atenolol	Anxiety management Cognitive therapy Social skills training
Obsessive-compulsive disorder	Clomipramine Fluoxetine Fluvoxamine	Exposure plus response prevention Thought stopping
Post-traumatic stress disorder	Imipramine Phenelzine	Psychotherapy Systematic desensitization

of panic attacks (Noyes et al., 1989b). About 20 percent experience an overstimulatory response to the initial doses of imipramine. This reaction is often quite unpleasant, leading patients to discontinue the drug unless warned in advance of its occurrence. Because many patients are sensitive to the side effects and react with increased anxiety initially, the drug should be started at 25 mg at bedtime and increased by 25 mg every third day as tolerated. Patients who respond should continue the drug for six months to a year before gradually discontinuing it. In the meantime, a lower maintenance dose may be found (Noyes et al., 1989a). About one-third of these patients gain weight on imipramine. Other tricyclics appear to be effective, and drugs like desipramine and nortriptyline may be better tolerated.

Patients who fail to respond to imipramine should be switched to phenelzine (Noyes et al., 1986). This drug is very effective but, because of the need for a tyramine-free diet and the risk of hypertensive crises, it is usually reserved for patients who have failed to respond to other drugs. Fortunately, hypertensive crises are rare, but should such a crisis occur, a patient should go to the nearest emergency room to have the blood pressure brought down. Patients should receive at least 60 mg daily for six weeks before concluding that the drug is ineffective. Postural hypotension and initial insomnia are sometimes troublesome side effects, and weight gain may occur later on. Tranylcypramine is less likely to produce postural hypotension and weight gain (Sheehan et al., 1980–81).

In controlled studies, alprazolam has been shown to be effective and well tolerated for panic disorder (Ballenger et al., 1988). In doses of up to 6 mg daily, the drug frees the majority of patients from panic attacks. Sedation, when it occurs, usually subsides in a few days or responds to a reduction in dose. The drug should not be given to patients who have a history of alcohol or drug abuse. Nor should it be given without warning patients of its habit-forming potential (Noyes et al., 1988). Because the response to the drug is rapid, it is useful for achieving prompt control of symptoms before a tricyclic antidepressant has taken effect. To avoid rebound or withdrawal symptoms, the drug should be discontinued gradually at a rate of no more than 0.5 mg every three or four days; also, if the patient is taking less than 2 mg daily, the rate should be 0.25 every three or four days. Other benzodiazepines such as diazepam, lorazepam, and clonazepam, appear to work just as well. Patients who experience inter-dose rebound with alprazolam may be switched to the longer-acting clonazepam. (Alprazolam, 1.0 mg, is roughly equivalent to clonazepam, 0.5 mg.)

Behavior therapy appears to be effective for panic disorder even when no phobic avoidance is present (Table 9–1). However, because few studies have been published, the efficacy of this approach relative to pharmacological treatments is not known, and its role in the overall treatment of panic disorder remains unclear. Somatic sensations such as dizziness or palpitations often appear to set off an anxious response. With this in mind, patients are taught to reproduce such sensations by hyperventilation, exercise, or some other means so as to desensitize themselves to triggers of panic. In 5 one-hour sessions, Barlow and Cerny (1988) also train patients to relax, to modify catastrophic thinking, to breathe in a measured fashion, and to expose themselves to external (phobic) stimuli where appropriate. These authors claim that their approach eliminates panic attacks and is as effective in this regard as drug therapy. Also, Beck's cognitive therapy may be effective by itself (Beck et al., 1985).

Agoraphobia

Patients with panic disorder who have phobic avoidance or agoraphobia should receive exposure in vivo regardless of whether they are given a drug to control panic attacks (Marks and Horder, 1987). Studies have shown that this is the most effective behavioral intervention and that it works in 60 to 75 percent of patients. In its simplest form, it consists of therapists' instructions to patients to challenge themselves in phobic situations until they are able to enter these situations without discomfort. Some patients respond to this therapy alone. The remainder require therapist supervision of practice sessions in which patients expose themselves to progressively more difficult situations. Therapists need not accompany their patients, but a spouse or friend may do so and provide support. Panic attacks also respond to exposure in vivo. Cognitive therapy may be effective with agoraphobic patients as well (Beck et al., 1985). Because behavior and drug therapies interact positively, they should usually be administered together (Mavissakalian, 1988).

Simple Phobia

The treatment of choice for simple phobia is exposure in vivo. So far, drugs have been shown to be ineffective in treating this type of phobic disturbance (Noyes et al., 1986). In fact, when benzodiazepines or alcohol have been administered during exposure in treatment sessions, they have made phobic situations easier to confront but have led to a less favorable treatment response (Chambles et al., 1979). Exposure in vivo appears to be more effective than desensitization, although a variety of modifications in technique may be useful (Marshall and Segal, 1988). For example, participant modeling may enhance the response to exposure. With this strategy the therapist enters the phobic situation, after which the patient is encouraged to do the same. Many simple phobic patients respond to exposure in six or fewer sessions.

Social Phobia

The choice of treatment for social phobia depends upon the subtype of the disorder (Table 9–1) (Liebowitz et al., 1985). The generalized form, involving most social gatherings or encounters, is highly responsive to the monoamine oxidase inhibitor phenelzine. One of the first controlled studies of drug treatment for social phobia has established this as an effective agent in doses of 45 to 90 mg daily (Liebowitz, 1987). Not only does the drug reduce anxiety in social settings, but it also improves social functioning. Avoidant personality traits that many social phobics manifest are favorably modified so that patients become more outgoing and begin to interact meaningfully with others. Experts believe that tricyclic antidepressants are ineffective, although they have not been properly tested.

Social phobics, whose problems are circumscribed or limited to a single social situation such as speaking in public, may respond to the beta-adrenergic blocking drug atenolol (Liebowitz, 1987). Actually, beta-blocking drugs have been used for some time in single doses to reduce troublesome performance anxiety. Propranalol, in a dose of 10 to 40 mg taken one hour before an examination or performance, may reduce the subjective distress caused by the situation and, perhaps, even improve performance. Somatic symptoms such as palpitations and tremor are readily controlled by beta blockers and are often the targets of such therapy (Noyes, 1988b). Patients who have frequent contact with phobic situations may benefit from continuous administration of a beta-blocking drug. Atenolol, which does not cross the blood-brain barrier easily, has the advantage of having fewer central nervous system side effects. Also, because the drug is long-acting, a dose of 50 to 100 mg may be taken just once daily.

Alprazolam appears to be effective in reducing social phobic symptoms as well as avoidant personality traits (Reich and Yates, 1988). However, because of the risk of dependence in these patients and their tendency to use the drug before confronting phobic situations, this and other benzodiazepines should be used sparingly.

Two behavioral strategies, corresponding to contrasting theories about the fundamental disturbance in social phobia, have been employed in this disorder. Anxiety management training aims at reducing the anxiety that is believed to be the basis of the distress and dysfunction in social settings (Marshall and Segal, 1988). This training usually involves exposure to phobic situations, although arranging for real-life exposure to specific social settings may be difficult. Here substitutes may be available, such as toastmasters' clubs and therapy groups, or exposure in imagination may be undertaken. Some form of cognitive restructuring is also utilized to reduce the perceived consequences of physiological (e.g., sweating, blushing) or other dysfunctions and to replace negative expectations with positive ones. A number of other techniques such as relaxation training, exposure to internal cues, and distraction may also be part of a behavioral package (Liebowitz, 1987).

Social skills training may be of value for patients who appear deficient in this area (Marshall and Segal, 1988). In some instances, social phobic symptoms appear to result from awkwardness or ineptitude in social situations. Where this is the case, training in social skills may be of benefit.

Such training may be done in groups and usually focuses on developing assertiveness and communication skills. The latter involve learning to ask questions, paraphrasing what another person has said to keep conversations going, and expressing feelings to others. Public speaking skills may be improved with the help of a toastmasters' club. As with other disorders, drug and behavioral treatments should usually be combined.

Obsessive-Compulsive Disorder

The current drug of choice for obsessive-compulsive disorder is clomipramine, as shown in Table 9–1 (Jenike, 1985). This drug has recently become available in the United States. In a controlled multicenter trial, about one-half of the patients responded to the drug with substantial reductions in obsessions and compulsions (De Veaugh-Geiss et al., 1989). The therapeutic dose range for this drug is considered to be 150 to 300 mg daily. However, because of an increased risk of seizures in higher doses (roughly 2 percent at 300 mg or more daily), it is recommended that the dose be kept as low as possible and not exceed 250 mg daily. The side effects of this drug, including lethargy, weight gain, and sexual dysfunction, are poorly tolerated by some patients.

Clomipramine has proven superior to other tricyclic antidepressants in comparative trials. Even so, drugs like imipramine are occasionally effective, and the response to an individual drug may be difficult to predict. Although Marks (1983) believes that clomipramine is of little value in patients who are not depressed, the evidence for a primary antiobsessional effect is convincing. Even when patients respond, however, they usually have residual symptoms and, when the drug is discontinued, they tend to relapse. For the present, patients are encouraged to take clomipramine for six months before attempting to stop using it. If symptoms return, they may restart the medication at the lowest effective dose.

Fluvoxamine, a potent serotonin reuptake blocking drug, has shown promise in early trials as an antiobsessional agent. In one controlled study, fluvoxamine, in a range of 150 to 300 mg daily, led to improvement in 80 percent of patients (Perse et al., 1987). Unfortunately, this drug is not available in the United States, but a similar agent, fluoxetine, may be useful in obsessive-compulsive disorder. This drug may also be tolerated better than clomipramine. The effective dose for obsessive-compulsive disorder appears to be 60 to 100 mg daily. Monoamine oxidase inhibitors, such as phenelzine, may also be effective in certain patients. Trazodone is another agent that may sometimes be beneficial.

Behavior therapy leads to substantial improvement in 70 percent of patients with obsessive-compulsive disorder and should be part of the treatment for most patients. Exposure plus response prevention is the most effective technique; however, exposure alone is of little value (Foa et al., 1985). Depressed patients do not respond well and should receive an antidepressant before behavior therapy is begun. Also, patients who regard their obsessional concerns as realistic do less well. Patients who have obsessions alone are usually not suitable for exposure. However, some of them will benefit from a simple technique called "thought stopping," especially after having improved with medication. Studies have shown that the results of exposure plus response prevention may be improved by prolonging the treatment and using participant modeling.

Generalized Anxiety Disorder

According to certain authorities, patients with generalized anxiety disorders that are encountered in family practice can be successfully treated without medication (see Chapter 2). Of course, most patients with this disturbance are, in fact, seen and treated by family practitioners. In this setting, the importance of communicating a specific diagnosis, offering reassurance about physical health, and providing education about anxiety disorders is very important (Noyes, 1987). Behavioral and cognitive strategies include relaxation training, breathing exercises, exposure to internal cues, distraction, and correction of cognitive distortions. Manuals for these simple techniques are widely available. Biofeedback and meditation may be employed as adjuncts. Also, where stressful life circumstances exist, supportive counseling may be helpful.

Diazepam continues to be a widely prescribed standard drug against which benzodiazepines are measured for the treatment of generalized anxiety. Other more potent agents, such as alprazolam, may be more effective but may have more dependence potential. Diazepam, in a range of 5 to 30 mg daily, not only reduces anxiety but also promotes sleep and muscle relaxation, both of which enhance its overall benefit. Studies suggest that while psychological dependence rarely develops, rebound anxiety occurs in a substantial minority of patients when benzodiazepines are discontinued. About one-half of long-term users experience withdrawal symptoms after abrupt discontinuation (Noyes et al., 1988). Drugs that are rapidly eliminated, such as lorazepam and alprazolam, are more apt to cause such problems. Dependence may be minimized by not prescribing benzodiazepines for patients who have histories of substance abuse and by administering them for brief periods of time.

Buspirone is a new benzodiazepine alternative. It is apparently free of addictive potential and has the further advantage of being nonsedating. However, questions have arisen about its effectiveness relative to the benzodiazepines, and it is known to have a delayed onset of action. The drug appears to have little value in treating benzodiazepine withdrawal. Tricyclic antidepressants also appear to be effective in generalized anxiety disorder. For example, imipramine was superior to chlodiazepoxide in one controlled trial (Kahn et al., 1986). Sedating tricyclics, such as doxepin and amitriptyline, are effective in low dose (i.e., 50 to 75 mg daily) and, like benzodiazepines, produce a response in one or two days.

Post-Traumatic Stress Disorder

Because post-traumatic stress disorder is caused by emotionally traumatic events or circumstances, many feel that the treatment of choice is
supportive or dynamically oriented psychotherapy (Table 9–1) (Hendin
and Haas, 1988). The psychotherapeutic approach to acute disturbances
began with the Pentothal-enhanced abreaction utilized during the Second
World War to restore psychiatric battlefield casualties to duty. Most interventions aim at helping patients to reexperience the traumatic event or
events and seek to restore their sense of mastery and meaning in life.
Behavior therapy is advocated for rape victims who suffer from post-
traumatic stress disorder. Most approaches combine systematic desensitization with cognitive restructuring and coping skills instruction (Foa et
al., in press). The objective of systematic desensitization, like that of psychotherapy, is to reduce the anxiety associated with situations or objects
that are not dangerous by the use of imagined exposure combined with
relaxation.

The drug that is perhaps most frequently prescribed is imipramine
(Frank et al., 1988). It appears capable of dampening the hyperarousal
associated with post-traumatic stress disorder and of reducing intrusive
recollections. Avoidant symptoms such as detachment and psychic numbing may not respond unless depression is also present (Friedman, 1988).
However, the antidepressant and antianxiety effects of imipramine may
lead to a beneficial reduction in common symptoms. This drug is relatively safe when drug or alcohol abuse is part of the picture. Sedating
tricyclics such as amitriptyline may be useful in promoting sleep as well
as in reducing daytime anxiety. Monoamine oxidase inhibitors, such as
phenelzine, are also useful in some cases of post-traumatic stress disorder. In addition to their antianxiety and antidepressant effects, these
drugs inhibit rapid eye movement sleep. Their stimulating effects may
help to interrupt the inertia and social withdrawal that are sometimes experienced by these patients. Monoamine oxidase inhibitors carry the risk
of hypertensive crises and require strict adherence to a tyramine-free diet.
Patients who abuse alcohol or drugs should not be given such medications. Benzodiazepines and beta blockers may also be effective with certain patients.

FUTURE DIRECTIONS

Evidence concerning the treatment of panic disorder suggests that combined drug and behavior therapies are most effective (Mavissakalian,
1988). This is likely to be the case for other anxiety disorders as well.
Therefore, what we need is more information about which patients are
likely to respond to which treatment combinations and how patients who
are less likely to respond to them can be identified. There is presently

little information about factors that predict a poor response. Also, continuing efforts must be made to determine which treatments are most cost effective. Some patients respond to simple education and instructions about self-directed exposure, while others require combinations of medication and therapist-assisted behavior therapy. Where treatment is offered, these options should be available and should involve appropriate professionals.

We must, of course, continue our search for new and more effective drugs and behavior therapies. Currently available drugs have a number of problems associated with their long-term use, and when they are withdrawn, relapse frequently occurs. We need more information in this area, but clearly, the value of medication is seriously reduced by these problems. Consequently, we must find ways of minimizing them through the development of safer, more effective agents and behavioral strategies that, when combined with drugs, enhance the effect of drugs and reduce the rate of relapse.

We need to develop strategies for treatment-resistant cases. This has been done for mood disorders, and some of the same measures, involving drug combinations, may prove useful for patients with anxiety disorders. The use of the controlled environment of the hospital for intensive medication and behavior therapies certainly needs further study (Pollard et al., 1987). Some of the treatment resistance that currently exists involves poor compliance. There are a variety of reasons for this, including the side effects of tricyclic antidepressants, but other factors, such as the attitudes of patients and their families, appear to be important as well and should be studied (Aronson et al., 1987).

There appear to be a number of reasons to encourage the development of anxiety disorder clinics where specialized treatment is made available. The prevalence of the anxiety disorders in the population should support such clinics in many communities. They make it possible to treat patients in groups, which is cost effective, and they also make a variety of therapists and therapies available that might not be found in more limited settings. Beyond this, they provide therapists with extensive experience, so that they become expert in managing anxiety disorders. Finally, they make sizable populations available for research protocols from which new treatment strategies may be developed and tested.

REFERENCES

Andrews G, Hadzi-Pavlovic D, Christensen H, et al: Views of practicing psychiatrists on the treatment of anxiety and somatoform disorders. *Am J Psychiatry* 144:1331–1334, 1987.

Aronson TA, Craig TJ, Thomason S, et al: Health care utilization patterns in panic disorder and agoraphobia. *J Anxiety Dis* 1:283–293, 1987.

Baer L, Minichiello WE: Behavior therapy for obsessive-compulsive disorder, in

Jenike MA, Baer L, Minichiello WE (eds): *Obsessive-Compulsive Disorders: Theory and Management*. Littleton, MA, PSG Publishing Co., 1986, pp. 45–76.

Ballenger JC, Burrows GD, DuPont RL, et al: Alprazolam in panic disorder and agoraphobia: Results from a multicenter trial. I. Efficacy in short term treatment. *Arch Gen Psychiatry* 45:413–422, 1988.

Barlow DH, Cerny JA: *Psychological Treatment of Panic*. New York, Guilford Press, 1988.

Beck AT, Emery G, Greenberg RL: *Anxiety Disorders and Phobias: A Cognitive Perspective*. New York, Basic Books, 1985.

Chambless DL, Foa EB, Groves GA, et al: Brevital in flooding with agoraphobics. *Behav Res Ther* 17:243–251, 1979.

Coryell W, Endicott J, Andreasen NC, et al: Depression and panic attacks: The significance of overlap as reflected in follow-up and family data. *Am J Psychiatry* 145:293–300, 1988.

De Veaugh-Geiss J, Landau P, Katz R: Treatment of obsessive compulsive disorder with clomipramine. *Psychiatr Ann* 19:97–101, 1989.

Diagnostic and Statistical Manual of Mental Disorders, ed 3 rev. Washington, DC, American Psychiatric Association, 1987.

Foa EB, Rothbaun BO, Steketee GS: Treatment of rape victims. NIMH Monograph Series, State of the Art Workshop on Sexual Assault, in press.

Foa EB, Steketee GS, Ozarow BJ: Behavior therapy with obsessive-compulsives: From theory to treatment, in Mavissakalian M, Turner SM, Michelson L (eds): *Obsessive-Compulsive Disorder: Psychological and Pharmacological Treatment*. New York, Plenum Press, 1985, pp 49–130.

Frank JB, Kosten TR, Giller EL, et al: A randomized clinical trial of phenelzine and imipramine for posttraumatic stress disorder. *Am J Psychiatry* 145:1289–1291, 1988.

Friedman MJ: Toward rational phramcotherapy for posttraumatic stress disorder: An interim report. *Am J Psychiatry* 145:281–285, 1988.

Hendin H, Haas AP. Post-traumatic stress disorder, in Last CG, Hersen M (eds): *Handbook of Anxiety Disorder*. New York, Pergamon Press, 1988, pp 127–142.

Jenike MA: Somatic treatments, in Mavissakalian M, Turner SM, Michelson L (eds): *Obsessive-Compulsive Disorders: Psychological and Pharmacological Treatment*. New York, Plenum Press, 1985, pp 77–112.

Jenike MA: Psychotherapy of the obsessional patient, in Jenike MA, Baer L, Minichiello WE (eds): *Obsessive Compulsive Disorders, Theory and Management*. Littleton, MA, PSG Publishing Co, 1986, pp 113–124.

Kahn RJ, McNair DM, Lipman RS, et al: Imipramine and chlordiazepoxide in depressive and anxiety disorders. II. Efficacy in anxious outpatients. *Arch Gen Psychiatry* 43:79–85, 1986.

Lelliott PT, Marks IM, Monteiro WO, et al: Agoraphobics five years after imipramine and exposure: Outcome and predictors. *J Nerv Ment Dis* 175:599–605, 1987.

Liebowitz MR: Social phobia. *Mod Prob Pharmacopsychiat* 22:141–173, 1987.

Liebowitz MR, Gorman JM, Fyer AJ, et al: Social phobia: Review of a neglected anxiety disorder. *Arch Gen Psychiatry* 42:729–736, 1985.

Marks IM: Are there anticompulsive or antiphobic drugs? Review of the evidence. *Br J Psychiatry* 143:338–347, 1983.

Marks IM, Horder J: Phobias and their treatment. *Br Med J* 295:589–591, 1987.

Marshall WL, Segal Z: Behavior therapy, in Last CG, Hersen M (eds): *Handbook of Anxiety Disorders*. New York, Pergamon Press, 1988, pp 338–361.

Mavissakalian MR: The mutually potentiating effects of imipramine and exposure in agoraphobia, in Hand I, Wittchen H (eds): *Panic and Phobias II: Treatments and Variables Affecting Course and Outcome.* Berlin, Springer-Verlag, 1988, pp 36–43.

Mavissakalian MR, Pevel JM: Imipramine dose–response relationship in panic disorder with agoraphobia. *Arch Gen Psychiatry* 46:127–131, 1989.

Mellman TA, Uhde TW: Obsessive-compulsive symptoms in panic disorder. *Am J Psychiatry* 144:1573–1576, 1987.

Noyes R: Is panic disorder a disease for the medical model? *Psychosomatics* 28:582–586, 1987.

Noyes R: Natural history of anxiety disorders, in Roth M, Burrows G, Noyes R (eds): *Handbook of Anxiety,* Vol. I. Amsterdam, Elsevier, 1988a, pp 115–133.

Noyes R: Beta-adrenergic blockers, in Last CG, Hersen M (eds): *Handbook of Anxiety Disorders.* New York, Pergamon Press 1988b, pp 445–459.

Noyes R: Revision of the DSM-III classification of anxiety disorders, in Roth M, Burrows G, Noyes R Jr (eds): *Handbook of Anxiety,* Vol. II. Amsterdam, Elsevier, pp 81–107, 1988c.

Noyes R, Chaudhry D, Domingo D: The pharmacological treatment of phobic disorders. *J Clin Psychiatry* 47:445–452, 1986.

Noyes R, Garvey MJ, Cook B, et al: Benzodiazepine withdrawal: A review of the evidence. *J Clin Psychiatry* 49:382–389, 1988.

Noyes R, Garvey MJ, Cook B, et al: Problems with tricylic antidepressants in patients with panic disorder: Results of a naturalistic follow-up study. J Clin Psychiatry, 50:163–169, 1989a.

Noyes R, Garvey MJ, Cook B: Follow-up study of patients with panic disorder and agoraphobia with panic attacks treated with tricyclic antidepressants. *J Affect Dis* 16:249–257, 1989b.

Perse TL, Greist JH, Jefferson JW, et al: Fluvoxamine treatment of obsessive-compulsive disorder. *Am J Psychiatry* 144:1543–1548, 1987.

Pollard CA, Obermeier HJ, Cox GL: Inpatient treatment of complicated agoraphobia and panic disorder. *Hosp Community Psychiatry* 38:951–958, 1987.

Reich J, Yates W: A pilot study of treatment of social phobia with alprazolam. *Am J Psychiatry* 145:590–594, 1988.

Ross HE, Glaser FB, Germanson T: The prevalence of psychiatric disorders in patients with alcohol and other drug problems. *Arch Gen Psychiatry* 45:1023–1031, 1988.

Sheehan DV, Claycomb JB, Kouretas N: Monoamine oxidase inhibitors: Prescription and patient management. *Int J Psychiatr Med* 10:99–121, 1980–81.

Stavrakaki C, Vargo B: The relationship of anxiety and depression: A review of the literature. *Br J Psychiatry* 149:7–16, 1986.

Zitrin CM, Klein DF, Woerner MG, et al: Treatment of phobias. I. Comparison of imipramine hydrochloride and placebo. *Arch Gen Psychiatry* 40:125–138, 1983.

Index